THE EAST INDIA COMPANY
AND
MEDICINE IN INDIA

The East India Company

and

Medicine in India

T. J. S. Patterson MD FRCS

SERENDIPITY

Copyright © T. J. S. Patterson 2007

First published in 2007 by

Serendipity Publishers, Darlington, UK

All rights reserved
Unauthorised duplication
contravenes existing laws
British Library Cataloguing-in-Publication data
A catalogue record for this book is available from the British Library

ISBN 978-1-84394-214-6

To the memory of the late Professor D.V. Subba Reddy (1899-1986),
doyen of historians of Medicine in India.

CONTENTS

ACKNOWLEDGEMENTS	viii
PREFACE	ix

I – INTRODUCTION

1
1 The spice trade and the early traders	5
2 Indian Medicine	

II – THE ESTABLISHMENT OF THE EAST INDIA COMPANY IN INDIA 1600-80

3 Founding the Company and training the surgeons.	19
4 The early voyages (1601-23)	29
5 Arrival in India	43
6 Acclimatization	59

III – THE RISING POWER OF THE COMPANY 1680-1780

7 Increasing medical experience	77
8 War with the French	101
9 The end of the Mogul Empire	127

IV – ORIENTALISM 1780-1835

10 Reforms in India	147
11 Renewed interest in Indian Medicine	167

V – WESTERNIZATION 1835-58

12 Establishment of western ('modern') medicine	185
13 The end of Company rule	203

VI – MEDICINE IN INDIA AFTER 1858

14 The role of the Indian Medical Service	215
15 The revival of Indian Medicine	225
16 Independence	231

EPILOGUE	237
APPENDIX – Botany and drugs in India	239
BIBLIOGRAPHY	253
INDEX	263

ACKNOWLEDGEMENTS

I am grateful for financial support from the E. P. Abraham Cephalosporin Fund, and from the Wellcome Trust to enable me to study in India.

In the Wellcome Unit for the History of Medicine in Oxford I had the advice and support of Charles Webster, Margaret Pelling and many other colleagues. Emilie Savage-Smith and Michael Dols helped my understanding of Islamic medicine.

I would like to thank the Directors and staff of the libraries I have consulted – the Bodleian, particularly the Indian Institute Library and the Radcliffe Science Library, the India Office Library and Records, and, in India, the National Archives (Delhi), the Tamil Nadu State Archives, the libraries of Osmania Medical College (Hyderabad), the Asiatic Society (Calcutta), Banaras Hindu University (Varanasi), the All-India Institute of Medical Sciences (Delhi), the Institute for History of Medicine at Tughlaqabad (with generous hospitality from Hakeem Abdul Hameed) and the Asiatic Society of Bombay.

By courtesy of the executors of the late Colonel H. W. Mulligan, CMG, IMS, I have been able to consult his (unpublished) *Facets of Research in British India by the Indian Medical Service 1600-1947.*

PREFACE

'It was settled by general consent that India was quite a misrepresented country, and had nothing objectionable in it, but a tiger or two, and a little heat in the warm part of the day.'

David Copperfield

The European Companies trading to the East – Portuguese, 1510; Dutch, 1596; English, 1601; French, 1668 – were set up to capture a share of the very lucrative spice trade. The English (later the British) East India Company, starting from a few small scattered factories (trading posts) in the East Indies and India, became the largest and most powerful trading company in the East. By the beginning of the nineteenth century it was the effective government of British India, although still technically a company of traders who were 'servants' under the authority of a Court of Directors in London. After the Indian Mutiny[1] in 1857 the Company's powers were transferred to the Crown in 'An Act for the better Government of India' (1858).

Apart from a few isolated travellers and missionaries, the Portuguese, at the beginning of the sixteenth century, were the first to bring European medicine to India. There they came in contact with the classical Indian medical systems, Ayurveda (Hindu) and Unani (Muslim), which had been highly developed (Ayurveda particularly in surgery) at a much earlier period. The traders, at first, did not distinguish these classical systems from the folk-medicine that was widespread in coastal and rural areas.

Each trading company brought its own surgeons with their contemporary medical practice. From its first expedition (1601) the English Company always had some sort of medical service. Every ship setting out for the East carried surgeons, and some of them remained on land with the early settlements. But they had little experience of tropical diseases which were either unknown or presented as familiar diseases in unexpectedly virulent forms. Their drugs and methods of treatment were often useless or actually harmful. They noted the work of Indian practitioners, and they were ready to learn how to use local drugs and techniques. Later, Indians would adopt some of the European methods. This interaction of western medicine[2] and Indian Medicine has continued up to the present.

As the power of the Company increased towards the end of the seventeenth century the earlier dependence on Indian Medicine was replaced by the criticism that it had remained unchanged for centuries. This 'stagnant' state of Indian Medicine was condemned by successive generations of Company surgeons who brought with them the more scientific medicine that was being developed in Europe.

From the 1740s the Company was involved in war with the French in India to protect its trading interests. Large armies were formed in the three Presidencies – Bengal, Madras and Bombay – and the French were finally defeated in 1761. The Company's medical services were put on a regular footing, and in 1764 all the medical officers in Bengal were organized into the Bengal Medical Service,[3] followed by similar arrangements in Madras and Bombay. In 1897 these were amalgamated into the Indian Medical Service which continued until Independence in 1947.

During the whole of this period the relation of western medicine to Indian Medicine varied with the changing military and political activities of the Company, and with developments in medicine in Europe.

Towards the end of the eighteenth century the Enlightenment in Europe was reflected in India by a general interest in Indian culture and science, including medicine. The earlier criticisms were replaced by renewed study of Indian Medicine and regular consultation with its practitioners. Company medical officers began to train Indian doctors, at first partly in western medicine and partly in Indian Medicine in the vernaculars. The Indian operation to replace missing parts of the face was witnessed and copied by Company surgeons. They transmitted the technique to London, and it was the starting point for the modern specialty of plastic and reconstructive surgery.

In the early nineteenth century these liberal 'orientalist' views were overtaken by the rise of imperialism and the policy of 'westernization'. English became the official language, and all support for Indian Medicine was withdrawn. The influence of the Company's medical officers now ensured that western medicine was widely practised, and that only western medicine was taught to the increasing numbers of Indians in the medical schools. The Company was thus responsible for the establishment of modern medicine in India.

After the end of Company rule (1858), the Indian Medical Service brought about major advances in tropical medicine, but these were mainly to protect the health of the military and of civilians in urban areas. Many of the village people were left to the care of Indian practitioners. Teaching of Indian Medicine was now largely confined within the family, handed down from father to son unchanged from the classical authors of fifteen hundred years before.

From the 1920s the growth of Indian nationalism brought increased status to Indian Medicine. Since Independence (1947), with official support, it is running in parallel with 'modern' medicine.

Notes

1 The Sepoy Rebellion, as it is known in India.

2 Called 'modern' medicine in India today.

3 The formation of the Bengal Medical Service was taken by its members as the date of origin of the Indian Medical Service.

THE EARLY VOYAGES (1601-23)

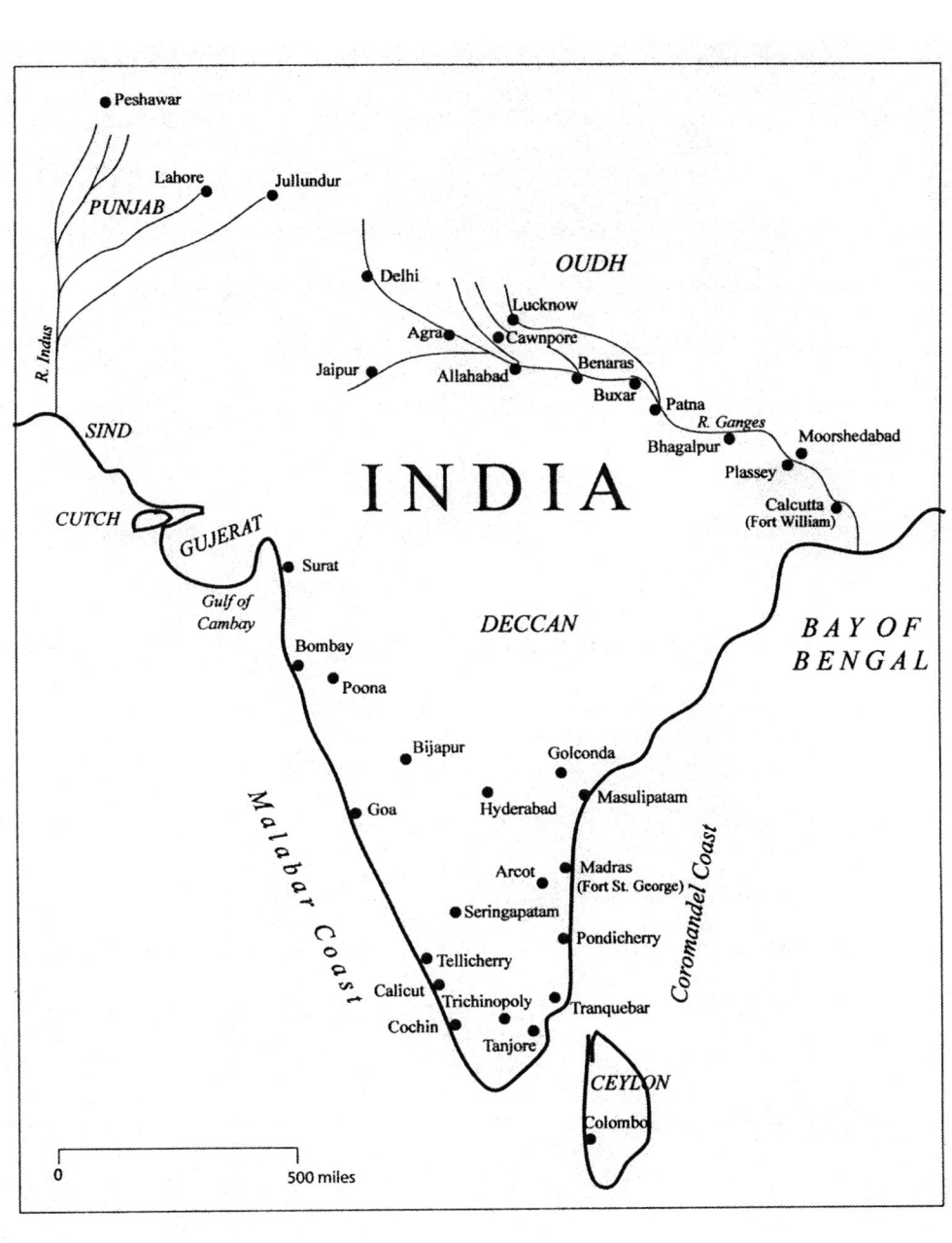

I
INTRODUCTION

Chapter One
The spice trade and the early traders

From early Roman times there was a demand in Europe for spices from the East. Spices were difficult to obtain and therefore expensive. It was a sign of wealth and status to have a constant supply. For the merchants they were light and compact to transport and very profitable. In northern Europe in the sixteenth century they were essential, for those who could afford them, for preserving food, overcoming the monotony of the diet, and disguising the flavour of tainted or salted meat.[1]

Cargoes of spices had always included medicinal substances. Galen, in Rome c. AD 180, had prescribed drugs from India. In the seventeenth century opium, nux vomica (strychnine), rhubarb, ginger and camphor were highly valued. Any new remedies for syphilis, such as sarsaparilla and China Root, were of particular interest (p.93).

Nearly all spices were also used as drugs. Pepper, which was most in demand for its flavour and for pickling meat, was regularly prescribed for diseases of the eye. Cinnamon was used for flavouring and its bark as a purge. There were also previously unknown plants with reputed medicinal properties which were imported for possible cultivation in Europe.

India was the intermediary in the Roman trade with the East, the goods being carried by sea to the mouth of the Red Sea and then on to the Mediterranean by caravan. From the seventh century AD Arabs began to play an increasingly important part, and up to the end of the fifteenth century the spice trade was in their hands, with Venice as the centre for distribution in Europe.

From the beginning of the sixteenth century the continuing demand for spices, and the large profits to be made, encouraged European traders to sail directly for the spice markets in the East. They headed for the Spice Islands, and they regarded India as a staging post. They followed the pattern established by the Arabs, reaching India on the summer monsoon,[2] continuing on to the East Indies and the Spice Islands, and timing their return to India to pick up the north-east wind. The round-trip often took up to three years.

The Portuguese were the first to reach India. From the middle of the fifteenth century they had been sending expeditions on short voyages along the west coast of Africa, and in 1487 Bartholomew Diaz rounded the Cape. In 1493 the Pope decreed that all new lands were to be divided between Spain and Portugal – Spain taking all to the west, and Portugal those to the east. Vasco da Gama founded the first settlement in India at Calicut on the Malabar (west) Coast in 1498. By 1510 they were firmly established along the west coast with their capital at Goa. By 1517 they had reached Canton in South China. Their vast area of influence was controlled from Goa – 'the Golden Age of Goa' (1510-c.1625). Like all the early traders, their power was at sea. They were confined to the coastal areas, which they controlled from their forts, and they had little influence inland. They defeated the Arabs at sea, and Lisbon became the centre of the European spice trade. Distribution was controlled by the Dutch with their superior local shipping and the banking centre in Amsterdam.

After the union of Portugal and Spain under Philip II in 1580 and the revolt of the provinces of the Netherlands, the Dutch were forbidden further trading with Lisbon. This spurred them to set up their own expeditions. Their first voyage reached Bantam in Java in 1596 and made a profit of 2,500 per cent. The Dutch could out-fight the Portuguese at sea, but they were unable to gain control on land. By 1620 they had abandoned their attempts to settle in India, and had established the centre of their empire in the East Indies at Jakarta. Here their chief rivals were the English whose first expedition reached Achin in Sumatra in 1602 and established a factory (trading post) at Bantam in 1603. But the Dutch were always more powerful in the East Indies. The English struggled against them for some years, but were forced to withdraw in 1623 to concentrate on trade with Persia and India where they had set up a factory at Surat in 1608.

The French established a factory at Surat in 1668 and their main centre at Pondicherry in 1674. In the eighteenth century they were the rivals of the (now British) Company for territory and trading in India. There was continuous fighting from the 1740s. The French were finally defeated and Pondicherry surrendered in 1761 leaving the British in control of large areas of India.

The Danes formed a trading company in 1612, reaching India in 1616. Their settlements, part of the Protestant missions from the Kings of Denmark, were relatively small and scattered. The company was wound up and sold to the British in 1845.

All these early expeditions were at risk from storms, shipwreck and battles at sea, but a greater hazard of the long sea voyage was illness, particularly scurvy (p.32). The ships were often out of sight of land for several months and unable to pick up fresh fruit and vegetables. There was a high sickness- and death-rate, not only from the disease itself but from its predisposition to other diseases such as dysentery. On reaching land the crews and their passengers, already weakened, were exposed to new and virulent infections. There were further deaths, made all the more alarming by the rapid course of some of the diseases and by the loss of so many men from relatively small communities. They were short of surgeons and European drugs. Each ship carried one or more surgeons but they died at the same rate as their patients, and their drugs and stores had often been damaged or destroyed at sea. They had little experience of tropical diseases, and they knew nothing of Indian Medicine. They found that standard European remedies were useless, or even harmful, for Indian diseases, and they sought any medical help that was available. Confined at first to coastal areas, they encountered the folk-medicine that was the prevailing system in the villages, with its belief in the supernatural causes of disease which were treated by charms, herbal preparations and prayers, in much the same way as village-medicine in other parts of the world (p.14).

Later, as they moved further inland and into the cities, they learned of the two classical systems, Ayurveda (Hindu) and Unani (Muslim). Some aspects of these would have seemed familiar as both are based on the doctrine of humours, like European medicine in the sixteenth and early seventeenth centuries (p.13). But, at first, they made no distinction between the folk-medicine and the classical systems, assuming that the more bizarre practices of the former were common to all Indian Medicine.

But knowledge of Indian Medicine in Europe at that time was very limited. Interchange of medical and scientific information between Indians and Arabs trading along the west coast of India from the seventh century AD had led to translations of Hindu medical texts into Arabic. Arab practitioners of Islamic medicine in the ninth to eleventh centuries had a wide knowledge of Ayurveda which they incorporated into their writings. Translations of these into Latin in the thirteenth century, transmitted through Spain and North-West Africa, became standard medical texts in Europe in the Middle Ages.[3] In this way some Indian medical knowledge reached the West. But most of it remained unknown in Europe until the end of the eighteenth century when the first translations from the original Sanskrit were made (p.149). Only then was it appreciated how highly Indian Medicine had been developed at a much earlier time.

Notes

1 For lack of fodder, cattle had to be slaughtered in the autumn, and all meat for the winter was salted.

2 The regularity of the monsoon (an Arabic word) was well-known.
The south-west wind in summer brought the ships on to the west coast of India, with the north-east wind in winter for the return voyage.

3 Rhazes (865-925) *On smallpox and measles*; Albucasis (c. 960 in Cordoba) *On surgery*; Ibn Sina (Avicenna) (980-1037) *Canon of medicine*.

Chapter Two
Indian Medicine

Medicine in India started in the Indus Valley Civilization (the Harappan Culture) (2500-1500 BC). Excavations in what is now Pakistan have shown large well-planned cities with a brick-built system of public and private water-supply and drainage. The people (Dravidians) were expert potters and metal-workers living in an urban civilization. From about 1500 BC the Indus Valley was repeatedly invaded from the north-west by Vedic Aryans who were primarily agricultural. The Dravidians were driven out and finally reached South India. It has been suggested that they took their system of medicine (Siddha) with them,

Siddha is now practised in South India in areas where Tamil is spoken. It has many similarities with Ayurveda and the two are linked together as one system in Indian Medicine today.[1] There is debate about its antiquity, but it is particularly associated with the early use of metals in medicine and alchemy. There are no references to surgical instruments or operations in Siddha texts. Their medicine is primarily preventive, although there are many topical remedies for wounds and ulcers. Certain families have special skills in reducing fractures and dislocations and in treating fistulae and piles; their remedies are kept secret within the family.

The arts, crafts and religious practice of the Vedic Period (1500-500 BC) were codified in the four Vedas as summaries of oral teaching written in Sanskrit, the cultural language of the Hindus; this technique was established by 500 BC. The Vedic people believed in the natural and moral order of the world as controlled by the gods who also played a part in treating disease. Man was born in human or animal form according to his good or evil deeds in an earlier life; disease was linked with sin. All matter, including the human body, was made up of the five elements: earth, air, fire, water and aether. The Vedic texts are collections of sacred songs and rituals, and not books of medicine, but they contain some anatomical and physiological information. Many of the observations refer to animals such as the horse which was the main victim of Vedic sacrifices. There are descriptions of two of the three classical humours: 'wind' (*vata*) and 'fire' (*pitta*, bile). Treatment, both to ward off and to treat disease, was by hymns, prayers and magic ritual. These were combined with plant remedies and some minerals. Plants were classified by their medicinal properties.

By about 500 BC Vedic religion had changed into something that is today recognized as Hinduism although this term was not used until very much later. Vedic medical practice began to be codified into Ayurveda, the 'science of life' of the Hindus. Ayurveda, which is part of the fourth Veda (Atharvaveda), took over many of the Vedic concepts including the belief that life and health are controlled partly by *karma* (the good or evil done in this or former lives) and partly by a man's own efforts. But the functioning of the body is controlled by natural laws, and, except in a very few instances, diseases are not due to gods or demons. Ayurveda aims not only to cure disease but to maintain health and bring longevity by emphasis on diet and regimen adapted to the individual, his surroundings and the climate.

From the eleventh century AD there were repeated Muslim invasions of India from the north-west, culminating in the founding of the Mogul Empire by Babur in 1526, by which time the Portuguese were established on the west coast at Goa. The Muslims brought their Islamic system of medicine with them, known in India as Unani tibb.[2] This is Galen's Graeco-Roman system of humours in health and disease,[3] derived from the Hippocratic school. In the fourth to sixth centuries AD Greek scholars had moved, or were driven, into Persia taking Greek medical texts with them. Islamic/Muslim medicine was founded in the eighth and ninth centuries by translation of these into Arabic. Its authorities are the Islamic physicians of the ninth to eleventh centuries AD, particularly Rhazes, Albucasis and Avicenna (p.4). It was superimposed on the indigenous Bedouin medical tradition which had been sanctified by the Prophet and which held that diet was the best remedy for disease, although magical healing with prayers and amulets was always important.

In parallel with the two 'classical' systems and overlapping at many points was the folk-medicine that had existed since Vedic times, and is still deeply rooted in some village communities. Its practitioners always outnumbered the classical practitioners and were responsible for the treatment of the greater part of the population in rural areas. Disease was considered to have both natural causes (treated by physical remedies – herbs, oils, cauterization and diet) and, more commonly, supernatural causes (treated by exorcism and religious ceremonies); these measures were often combined. Villages were thought to be surrounded by evil spirits which had to be propitiated, often by animal sacrifice, to ward off epidemics and other misfortunes such as failure of the crops. Epidemics were explained as the wrath of a malevolent god or goddess, such as Sitala in smallpox (p.91).

There are similarities between folk- and classical Indian Medicine, and they were often confused by the early traders. The superstitious basis of folk-medicine and its lack of a written tradition led many of the English, towards the end of the seventeenth century, to regard all Indian Medicine as quackery.

Ayurveda has come down through two main schools: Caraka of Kashmir, mainly concerned with internal medicine, and Susruta of Benares (Varanasi) which covers internal medicine, but adds large sections on the teaching and practice of surgery. Susruta is claimed in India today as 'the father of surgery'. The dating of Indian manuscripts is often uncertain, and it is made more complicated by confusion over authors' names, but the oldest surviving texts were probably written 200 BC – AD 200. Ayurveda deals with general medicine, mental disorders, children (with childbirth and diseases of women), surgery, diseases of the eye, ear, nose and throat, poisons (including snake-bite), rejuvenation and longevity, and fertility and virility. There are also sections concerned with animals (particularly the cow, horse and elephant), and with trees and plants. Susruta regards surgery as the most important part, as it can bring quick cures.

The doctrine of Ayurveda follows the Vedic concept of the five elements which make up all the tissues of the body. The elements act in the body in the form of three humours (*dos(h)as*) (the first two were already part of Vedic thought): *vata* (wind/breath/air), concerned with all movements; *pitta* (bile/fire) cooks the food, colours the blood, excites desires and gives sight; and *kapha* (phlegm/mucus/water) connects all the parts together, supports the heart, and gives sensation in the head. Blood is recognized as a vital factor in disease, but is not regarded as a fourth humour (as in Unani). The proportions of the three humours vary from person to person. Their actions vary according to the season, the environment, the life-style of the individual, and his diet. In good health they are in equilibrium; disease results from their imbalance. The seasons have important effects, and the physician is required to take the appropriate preventive measures in each season.

There were high standards of training which took seven to eight years. The teacher repeated verses of the text until the student had learned them by heart; the teacher then explained and elaborated them. The verses were very compressed, but it has been calculated that the student would have had to learn twelve *slokas* (of thirty-two syllables each) every day for eight years, allowing forty-eight days holiday each year. The student was urged to learn as much as he could from the herdsmen and men of the forest and hills who would all have good knowledge of the herbs in their neighbourhood. Knowledge of anatomy was obtained by wrapping cadavers in grass, and suspending them in a cage in a slowly-flowing river for seven days. They were then dissected by rubbing off the outer layers with brushes. The bones were fairly accurately described, but knowledge of the muscles and vessels was rudimentary. Little was known about the brain and the lungs, but organs such as the rectum, bladder and vagina, which were familiar from surgical manipulations, were carefully described. The circulation of the blood was not understood; venous blood was thought to be converted into arterial in the liver. The heart was, at first, the central organ of consciousness; later this was transferred to the brain and spinal cord.

There was practical training in medical procedures: removal of disordered humours by emetics, purging, enemas, sweating and blood-letting, or specifically from the head by inhalations, snuffs and gargles. Surgical techniques were practised on inanimate objects: puncturing lotus stalks, probing a dried gourd, suturing pieces of soft leather. The use of the cautery and caustics was also taught.

After periodic tests and a final examination viva voce, the student was bound to his teacher at a solemn ceremony with an address on medical ethics. The teacher was made responsible for the student in his future practice. The qualified Ayurvedic physician was known as vaidya ('knowledge'). Vaidyas were highly regarded by the King, and they were expected to be in constant attendance, particularly when he was on the move with his army. The detection and treatment of poisoning was an important part of their duties. They were in charge of the kitchens to control the King's diet and prevent him and his men being poisoned. The Ayurvedic texts give detailed descriptions of organic and inorganic poisons and of poisoning by the bites of snakes, scorpions, spiders, rats and rabid animals. Prognosis – forecasting the outcome of a disease – was a particularly important part of the vaidya's practice. He had to be able to recognize incurable disease, because this was not to be treated.[4]

The aim of Ayurveda is to maintain health and bring longevity by diet and a regime that will prevent imbalance of the humours, adapted to the individual, his mental state, his living conditions and the season. Since diet is the basis of health, the physician must know the properties of all foodstuffs. The regime includes advice on cleansing the body, on exercise, sleep, sexual activity, and general ethical principles: politeness, obedience, honesty and devotion to the gods and the brahmins.

The treatment of disease is determined by the humour or humours that are disturbed (aggravated or vitiated), and is designed to restore the balance. Drugs are prescribed that have a soothing or stimulating effect as necessary. Ayurveda is thus, like western medicine, allopathic (a disease is cured by its opposite or antidote), in contrast to homoeopathy ('like cures like').

At first mainly vegetable materials were used, each preparation usually consisting of multiple ingredients. Susruta gives a list of nearly 500 medicinal herbs. Aphrodisiacs were important among the measures to retain virility and ensure a long life. There were none of the later taboos on animal products or alcohol; the stages and management of drunkenness were described. Later, minerals were introduced, based on earlier alchemical practices (p.12). Among the remedies for venereal diseases were metallic preparations – iron and copper, but not mercury,

Fasting was an important part of many of the treatments, particularly for fevers and diarrhoea and allied disorders. This was combined with specific drugs and emetics, purges and enemas (the best for all diseases) to remove vitiated humours. In severe cases of diarrhoea when the patient was semi-conscious (probably cholera) red-hot cautery was applied to the soles of the feet.

A disease known as 'honey-urine' (which would now be recognized as diabetes) was accurately described. Leprosy was recognized and distinguished from patchy depigmentation of the skin (p.168). Although it might prove to be incurable, treatment was urged to prevent it persisting into the next life. Among the recommended remedies was tuvaraka (*Hydnocarpus laurifolia*).[5]

Treatment generally excluded magic; the influence of demons was only postulated for madness and fits and some diseases of children. Religious ceremonies were part of some treatments, particularly in connection with childbirth and surgical operations.

Surgery in Ayurveda reached a higher standard than in any other early system of medicine. A wide range of operations was carried out with skilfully-made instruments, some of them of tempered steel. There were 101 blunt instruments and 20 sharp instruments. The student was trained in eight surgical procedures – excision, incision, scraping, puncturing, probing, extraction, drainage and suturing. Operations were carried out at an auspicious time, after prayers and offerings to the gods. The patient was placed facing east, with the surgeon facing west. Cannabis and other drugs to alter consciousness were well-known. Alcohol for the relief of pain was specifically mentioned by Susruta. Hymns against evil spirits were recited twice a day.

There were detailed instructions for the removal of foreign bodies, such as arrow-heads, and for the treatment of abscesses, piles, and fractures and dislocations. Stones in the bladder were removed by low lithotomy – opening the bladder from below and extracting the stone with a hook.[6]

Blockage in the guts was only to be treated after permission from the King. The belly was opened and the foreign body removed by cutting into the gut. The opening in the gut was closed by getting black ants to bite the edges together; their bodies were then pulled off, leaving the heads in place.[7]

Missing parts of the nose and the lobe of the ear were reconstructed by grafting a flap of skin from the adjoining cheek. For the nose, a leaf the size of the defect was used as a pattern on the cheek. A flap of skin of the same size was raised, keeping a partial attachment to the cheek for its nourishment, and stitched into place over two little tubes to keep the nostrils open.[8] A surgeon who could carry out these operations and also repair a hare-lip was fit to attend the King.

Blood-letting by venesection was used for quick relief of symptoms. It was as important a part of surgery as the enema in internal medicine. For more gradual withdrawal of blood, leeches were applied, or cupping after scarification.

Alkaline caustics were used to remove surface lesions, or, smeared on threads, introduced into the track to obliterate fistula-in-ano.[9] The actual cautery was used on all parts of the body to treat pain and to control bleeding. The areas were then dressed with honey and ghee (clarified butter).

Diseases of the eye were an important part of Ayurveda; the anatomy was accurately described. Many surgical procedures were used, including 'couching' for cataract, described in detail by Susruta.[10]

Obstetrics was covered from conception to care in pregnancy and during and after delivery, with the management of threatened abortion and malpresentations. The care of the new-born emphasized the risk that they might be affected by demons if they were ill-treated.

Unani holds that all matter is composed of four elements: earth, air, fire and water, with four qualities: cold, dry, hot and wet. Food and drink, consisting of these elements and their qualities after digestion, are transformed into four humours: blood, yellow bile, black bile, and phlegm. Good health depends on their balance. The proportion of each humour varies with the individual, influenced by external factors such as climate, occupation and the season. One humour dominates in every human being, and determines the disposition: sanguine, choleric (bilious), melancholic, or phlegmatic. The physician's task is to preserve health and treat disease by a regimen that emphasizes diet. Purges, emetics and bleeding are important in correcting imbalance. Great attention is always paid to psychological factors and the management of melancholy and other mental disorders.

Treatment is allopathic, like Ayurveda, and prescriptions are also made up of multiple ingredients on the theory that these will potentiate each other and antagonize adverse side-effects. Unani physicians (hakims), at an early stage, developed skills in the use of metals and minerals for medical treatment, and these were later passed on to Ayurveda. Unani had at first a range of surgical operations, but this was more restricted than Ayurveda, relying more on the cautery than the knife. Opium and other drugs were used for the alleviation of pain but there is no record of any anaesthetic being used. Alcohol was forbidden. There was particular expertise in diseases of the eye, including couching for cataract. Muslim ophthalmic treatises, translated into Latin, remained the best in Europe until the early eighteenth century.

Even before the Muslim invasions, Hindu medicine had become relatively static, concerned only to maintain the classical traditions. The writings of medical authors, such as Vagbhata (c. AD 650) and Madhava (c. AD 700), were mostly commentaries on the texts of Caraka and Susruta, and did not add anything to their general principles. Surgical expertise had begun to decline from about 200 BC. Surgery, at first, had been practised by men of high status. But its prestige had fallen, and the craft passed down the social scale,[11] becoming a tradition of single techniques e.g. couching for cataract, or reconstruction of missing parts of the face, handed down in a particular family. These families, usually of relatively low caste, kept their work secret.

The reasons for this decline are debatable. With increasing rigidity of the caste system, brahmins (the priestly caste) who had been the original practitioners and teachers came to believe that contact with blood was defilement. The surgeon might think that his training allowed him to incur pollution without the need for purification but he became increasingly looked down on by brahmins. At this time, also, there was a rapid spread of Buddhism, with its tenet of non-violence. Buddhists preached against the pain of surgical operations. Their influence may have reduced the number of wars and the need for surgery.

Buddhism[12] had started as a revolt against Hinduism in the fifth century BC. It expanded rapidly in India under the Emperor Ashoka (279-236 BC) from the middle of the third century, and then spread to Ceylon, Tibet and the Far East. Buddhists encouraged the study of medicine and taught it in their monasteries. Some of the principal writers on medicine were Buddhists. The monks took this knowledge with them on their missionary travels.

Contacts with China were on a limited scale until the first century AD, but then increased in the fourth to eighth centuries when there were prolonged interchanges with many embassies and ambassadors from China to India. But the medical systems remained separate. Very little Chinese medicine came back to India. Acupuncture never became part of Indian Medicine, and there is no mention of it in the classical texts.[13]

From the ninth century there had been Indian physicians at the Arab courts; Arab physicians went to India to learn Indian science and medicine, and taught Greek science to the Indians. This introduction of Islamic medicine into India increased with the Muslim invasions from the eleventh century. Ayurveda and Unani already had much in common. Both are based on a humoral theory supported by authoritative texts. Health depends on the balance of humours in the body, and disease is the result of imbalance. Both are allopathic, using drugs which are opposite in quality to correct the balance, and they stress that their remedies do no harm. Both have particular expertise in diseases of the eye. The patient is treated as a whole in relation to his environment, the season, the climate and his natural constitution, not only to cure disease, but to improve his general health and prevent recurrence.

By the sixteenth century they had existed side-by-side long enough for there to have been a great deal of interchange. The Emperor Akbar, who reigned from 1556-1605, created a State in which there were equal opportunities for Hindus. This changed with his bigoted successors (particularly Aurangzeb after 1680). But in Akbar's time Hindus practised Unani, and Muslims

Ayurveda, and both were consulted by people of both religions, although high-caste Hindus could only be treated by Hindus. The vaidyas learned the hakims' skill in examination of the pulse as a diagnostic and prognostic tool. The hakims, to suit Indian conditions, took over some of the Ayurvedic methods and drugs.

Hakims had great expertise in the use of metals and minerals as drugs, and added many new preparations to the pharmacopoeia. Earlier, vaidyas and hakims had worked together in the hospitals, although these were now in decline.

The Muslims had been the first to set up hospitals in India. Hindu rulers were expected to protect their subjects and provide free medical care for the poor. This was a particular concern of the Emperor Ashoka (third century BC). There were designated buildings, but these were probably small rest-houses for travellers for temporary use only and not for the systematic treatment of disease. Some temples, particularly Buddhist monasteries, provided medical care of pilgrims and the sick. Endowment of hospitals by Muslims was part of their charitable work. After their arrival in India, well-organized hospitals were set up in all the larger towns. Treatment was free and admission was open to all classes. There was particular care for lunatics and all mental disorders. But by the early seventeenth century, with the general decline of Muslim medicine (p.14), the hospitals had been abandoned. When the English arrived on the west coast in 1608 the only 'hospitals' they found were run by Hindus, and solely for the care of animals (p.55).

Ayurvedic drugs are predominantly herbal. Since they decayed rapidly, there were attempts to transfer their properties to metals, principally mercury, to make them durable. From the eleventh century complicated processes were developed to 'treat' metals and minerals with medicinal plants. The ill effects of mercury were well-known, and eighteen separate treatments were required to make it safe for internal use. This work was carried out particularly in Tamil-speaking areas of South India, where Siddha medicine is practised (p.5). The processes were kept secret and have not been reproduced, although something similar continues today using mercury, sulphur, silica and other chemicals with a large number of plants.

The use of metals in medicine had developed from experience of alchemical processes. Alchemy had been studied in India continuously from the Vedic period in the search for 'perfection' and immortality. The elixir was cinnabar (mercuric sulphide), which may originally have come from China. Later, with Ayurveda, the requirements were virility and longevity. From the fourth century AD attention turned to transmutation of metals, seeking to transmute base metals into the 'perfect and everlasting' metal – gold. By the end of the sixteenth century there had been many advances in the knowledge of different metals, minerals and their compounds. But alchemy, although continuing in South India, did not develop further. In Europe, by contrast, it was the foundation for the science of chemistry. Alchemical ideas, transmitted in Arabic texts in the twelfth century, helped to direct research in Europe into the preparation of medicines. Paracelsus,[14] in the early sixteenth century, opposed the humoral theories of Galen by regarding the body as a chemical system which could therefore be treated and cured by inorganic remedies. He held that the purpose of alchemy was to make medicines – not gold. He used a mixture of salt with mercury and sulphur, similar to the Hindu preparations, and he knew of its origin in India, referring to the 'Yogis of India'.

Until the mid-seventeenth century, when the pattern of European medicine began to change from Galenism (p.6), Indian and European medicine had many features in common. They each had a philosophical basis which was codified in written texts. Ayurveda and Unani are 'humoral', as was European medicine in the sixteenth century; Ayurveda has three humours, European and Unani the four derived from Greek medicine. They are all allopathic – a disease is to be treated by its opposite or antidote.[15] Unani and European medicine followed Galen's practice which had undergone little change since the second century AD. In all three, treatment was directed mainly to the relief of symptoms, and remedies were compounded of multiple ingredients, mostly herbal. They all stressed the importance of diet and a healthy regimen in treating and warding off disease and promoting a long life. They all relied on examination of the pulse for diagnosis and prognosis.[16]

Both Ayurveda and Unani claim to be in the direct line of the origin of modern medicine – Unani as the direct descendant of Greek medicine, and Ayurveda by its incorporation into Arab medicine from the tenth century and its transmission by the Arabs to the West. Up to the end of the eighteenth century little was known in Europe of any original thought by Indians, e.g. in mathematics or medicine. It was assumed that all Indian ideas must have come from the Greeks. The early traders noted the concern of Hindus for animals and the hospitals set up for their welfare. When they learned of the Hindu doctrine of metempsychosis (transmigration of souls) the more educated among them recognized the similarity with Pythagoras's teaching, and assumed that this was evidence of the Greek influence.

The difficulty in dating Indian texts, and confusion over authors' names, make it impossible to be certain of the dates of the original ideas. The surviving Indian medical texts, although written later than the Greek, contain many Vedic concepts, suggesting that the ideas originated earlier, and that there was a continuous tradition even though the intermediate texts have been lost. There are similarities in Greek and Indian Medicine. Hippocrates had the general concept of 'breath' or 'wind' as the motor force in the world and in the individual, and he recorded Indian medical remedies. It is possible that there were early exchanges of medical information between Greece and

India along the trade-route across Persia, and that the two medical systems developed in parallel.

By the time the English reached India, Ayurveda and Unani had been unchanged for many centuries, with their authorities still the classical texts. Hindu medical writings were often simply a list of prescriptions by physicians for their own use or for students. The most original writer in the sixteenth century was Bhavaprakasa who described syphilis (which, he said, had been introduced by the Portuguese) and its treatment with mercury.

The Indian Emperors who succeeded Akbar began to impose increased taxes and other repressive measures on Hindus, and they only gave official support to their own religion and science. Unani became the main practice in the cities and in the palaces and courts of noblemen. Ayurveda continued more in country districts and among the poor. Hindus began to keep their learning secret to protect it from Muslims.

But Muslim medicine was also declining as it came into conflict with increasingly conservative Islamic religious beliefs. The physician's practice was seen as incompatible with Islamic orthodoxy. There was very little operative surgery, but the actual cautery was widely used, for both humans and animals.

> Their horses are fine, but they have many distempers – mostly cured with a hot iron. 'Tis likewise the easiest and the fastest Cure for the Men of the East Country.

In both Europe and India folk-medicine was running in parallel with the classical systems. The supernatural causes of disease were still generally accepted by all classes of society, with the importance of magic, witchcraft and propitiation of the gods in prevention and cure. Both folk- and classical medicine were always in competition with the flourishing trade of itinerant quacks. Regular practitioners continually inveighed against them and tried to have them suppressed by legal sanctions.

The English would have found this pattern of medical practice familiar, although at first they did not distinguish between classical and folk-medicine in India. The university-educated physician, who might have appreciated the classical systems, was at that time thought to be unfitted for the rough-and-tumble of a trader's life. The first medical officers of the East India Company were all surgeons who had had a practical training as apprentices. With the decline of surgery in India their skills were soon in demand and would be exploited by the Company to promote goodwill in the interests of profitable trading.

Notes

1 The five systems that make up Indian Medicine are Ayurveda with Siddha (Hindu), Unani (Muslim), Homoeopathy (introduced into India c.1838), Naturopathy (favoured by Gandhi) and Yoga.

2 Unani means 'Greek' (correctly it should be Yunani; Unani is the English spelling); 'tibb' is the Arabic word for medicine. This term is only used in India and Pakistan.

3 Galen (c. AD 130-200) was a Greek physician who lived in Rome from the age of thirty. Most of the medical practice in Europe up to the early seventeenth century was based on his writings.

4 In the 1920s, in the debate on the revival of Indian Medicine, this principle of Ayurveda was regarded as unethical (p.227).

5 *Hydnocarpus* was the mainstay of treatment for leprosy in the nineteenth century and until the introduction of specific drugs in 1942 (p.222).

6 This was the standard technique in Europe until the nineteenth century. Samuel Pepys was successfully treated in this way on 26 March 1658.

7 Recent experiments have shown that this is a practicable technique.

8 This technique differs from that witnessed, and adopted, by Company surgeons towards the end of the eighteenth century, but both contributed to the development of the modern speciality of plastic and reconstructive surgery (p.172).

9 A discharging track opening internally in the rectum, and externally on the skin near the anus. Treatment with medicated threads is very effective, and is still used today, as demonstrated to the author at the Ayurvedic Hospital in Varanasi.

10 Couching (as with a lance) displaces the lens with a metal instrument. This was the standard operation in Europe, and continued in India into the nineteenth century (p.171); there was always a high rate of complications. This was the cause of Handel's blindness.

11 'Bleeding was left to the barbers, bone-setting to the herdsmen, and the application of blisters to every man.'

12 Buddha (born 586 BC) used the common language (Pali) in contrast to the Sanskrit of the brahmins.

13 The earliest report of acupuncture in India was in 1830 by F. H. Brett, a Company surgeon, who had learned the technique outside India (p.197).

14 Paracelsus (1493-1541), Swiss physician, led the revolt against Galen's herbal remedies, burning his works in Basle in 1527. His principles were followed particularly by surgeons in Europe. John Woodall, the first Surgeon-General of the East India Company (1612), was an enthusiastic paracelsian at a time when this was unpopular (p.21).

15 Homoeopathy – 'like cures like' – was founded by Samuel Hahnemann in Leipzig in the late eighteenth century and was introduced into India from Europe c. 1838 (p.225).

16 Pulse-lore, with its meticulous examination of one or both pulses, was still an important part of diagnosis in the early nineteenth century. Surgeon John Johnson, in 1815, discussing the diagnosis of liver disease, noted that 'the pulse, though neither hard nor very quick, will have an irritable throb, indicative of some internal affection'.

II
THE ESTABLISHMENT OF THE EAST INDIA COMPANY IN INDIA 1600-80

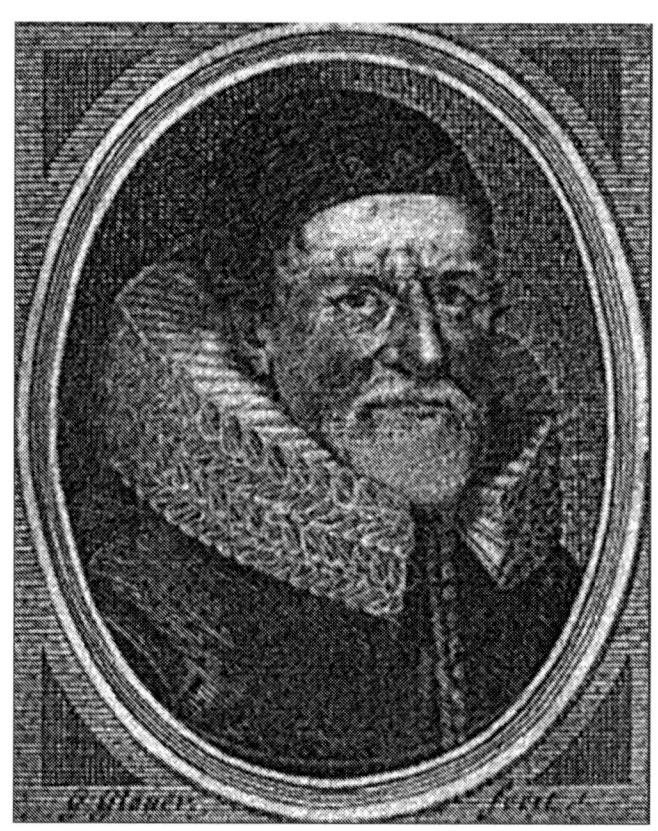

John Woodall (1570-1643), the first Surgeon-General of the East India Company (1612-43).

(Reproduced with permission from the Wellcome Library).

Chapter Three
Founding the Company and training the surgeons

From the last quarter of the sixteenth century London merchants had been making increasing efforts to break into the spice trade. Attempts to find a northern passage to the East were unsuccessful. The southern route was forbidden by Elizabeth for fear of offending Spain. Trading with India by land was expensive and already being undercut by the Dutch. The merchants sought a charter[1] that would give them the right to trade with the East by sea. Elizabeth's views began to change with the defeat of the Armada in 1588. After the death of Philip II in 1598 the merchants strengthened their case by appointing Richard Hakluyt as Historiographer to collect all the available information about trade with the East. In his report he gave a list of all the goods obtainable which included many 'spices' and 'drugs of all sorts'.

In 1600 another application was made as 'Certayne reasons why the English Merchants may trade into the East Indies, especially to such rich kingdoms and dominions as are not subjects to the Kinge of Spayne and Portugal'. This was accepted, and the first Charter was signed by Elizabeth on 31 December 1600 for 'The Governor and Company of Merchants of London trading into the East Indies'. This allowed them the rights of exclusive trade for fifteen years, and to purchase land without limit. They bought ships, and engaged 480 men. The complement for each ship included a merchant and 'Surgeons Twoe and a Barber'.

The title 'East India Company', often with the prefix 'Honourable' (HEIC), was used from the early times. At some time in the seventeenth century the name 'Jehan' or 'Jan' was introduced by the Dutch into their Company's title with the implication that there was a mighty Prince Jehan, with the surname 'Company', and that this would inspire more respect than that due to a band of traders. Later this was applied to the English Company – 'John Company' – a ruler who was never in India, but had his throne in London.

The Company was controlled by a Court of Directors with their headquarters in London. They were all strongly puritan, and they determined that the new Company would be made up of traders concerned only with making a profit for the Company, and that gentlemen-adventurers and noblemen would not be admitted. Their ruling was that 'freight is the mother of wages'. If a cargo was lost or damaged there would be deductions from the wages of the crew.

There was, at first, no organized medical service. Surgeons and mates (assistants) were recruited independently for a specific voyage or voyages. Some signed on for the round voyage only; others contracted for one or more tours of duty on land. They were examined in London by the Surgeon-General, the senior medical officer of the Company, who was also responsible for fitting out the surgeons' chests with drugs and instruments. From 1624 all applicants had to be approved by the Barber-Surgeons.[2] The university training of physicians was thought to make them unsuited to active service, and they were forbidden by law to serve the military. The Directors applied this principle to their early medical recruits who were all apprenticed surgeons or mates. The first physicians did not reach India officially until the end of the seventeenth century (p.81).

Although a certificated barber-surgeon might become very rich, the salaries offered to all Company 'servants', including surgeons, were relatively low. In 1615 a chaplain was paid £50 and a surgeon £24 per annum. In addition they were entitled to meals at the Common Table, and there were allowances for housing, servants, diet and liquor. Up to 1764 the surgeon's salary never rose above £36. He was allowed, and expected, to supplement this by private practice, and there were other sources of income, such as private trading and prize money. At first there were no pensions and no pay for injury or for dependents. Up to 1614 the Company dockyard was at Deptford with a resident surgeon whose room was used as a hospital; by 1618 the docks were employing 232 men. Then a new dock was opened at Blackwall which could hold three ships. The surgeon-in-charge attended the sick and injured, both in the docks and on the ships at anchor. He was also required to cut the men's hair; two pence per month was stopped from each man's wages to pay for this.

The first specific training for Company surgeons was given by John Woodall (1570-1643) who was already an experienced military surgeon by the time he was appointed Surgeon-General in 1612 (continuing until his death in 1643). In 1616 he was appointed surgeon to St Bartholomew's Hospital, and, in 1633, Master of the Barber-Surgeons Company. William Harvey was already a physician at St. Bartholomew's. Woodall was twenty-two years older than Harvey, but, as a Barber-Surgeon without knowledge of Latin, he was of inferior status. He was a widely-read man but he recognized the difference between an 'educated' physician and an 'experienced' surgeon. He pleaded for surgeons to be allowed to practise the whole of medicine and surgery, for they alone were responsible for the health of soldiers and sailors.[3]

In 1617 he published *The Surgion's Mate*[4] 'chiefly for the benefit of young Sea-Surgions, imployed in the East-India Companies affaires', the first manual for ships' surgeons. All the Company's ships and factories were supplied with copies. Much of his text was concerned with surgery, but he gave detailed information on the medical contents of the chest. He apologized to the 'learned' physicians for dealing with medicines so fully, but he only did it for the inexperienced young surgeon on his first voyage. The quality of his apprentices (from whom he took two months of their annual pay) was sometimes criticized – 'a man need only sleep under a medicine chest for a single night to become perfectly qualified for the office.' Woodall's reply was that no one else could be found to take such risks. By 1624 twenty of his pupils had died.

The young surgeon had to be competent to 'take a vaine smoothly and neate, as also to shave well is praise worthy'. He had to sharpen his own knives:

> it is a principall proofe-peece of mastership in Surgery, for a young man to take a base and ordinary knife, and to fit it to shave a beard.

He had to be expert at pulling teeth; a full set of dental instruments was provided. He was also the ship's barber, and there was a separate case with all the necessary equipment. This was carried with the other surgical instruments in the lid of the chest. If there was a shortage of instruments, the ship's carpenter could often supply what was needed.

Woodall gave detailed instructions for dealing with all conditions likely to be met at sea, with advice about the drugs and surgical instruments needed. He was, in general, a conservative surgeon and he continually urged this on his apprentices. The 'trapan' (trephine for opening the skull) that he had invented was to be used rarely and only after practice on a sheep's head. Knives 'are much less used amongst discreet Artists of our time, than it was in former ages'. Cauterizing irons also; they were terrifying for the patient, but they could be useful to control bleeding and for some cases of epilepsy and apoplexy. He warned that blood-letting should be carried out cautiously at sea, because the diet was often deficient, and 'in the blood consisteth the life of man'.

The body of the surgeon's chest contained a wide variety of vegetable and mineral drugs. Woodall was well aware of the problem of deterioration of drugs in a hot climate, and he preferred inorganic to herbal remedies for their keeping qualities although he warned of the dangers of overdosing with heavy metals, particularly mercury – 'for healing and killing Mercurie hath no fellow.' He quoted Paracelsus throughout this section (p.13). Of all the drugs, opium was the most important, and essential for a voyage to the East Indies. The best preparation was the *Laudanum Opiat Paracelsi* (tincture of opium), for 'many diseases and greefes, except when feeble with cough and sputum'. It had to be modified if given to women, but 'women in long voiages are rare creatures'.

For the 'flux' (diarrhoea, dysentery) his chief remedy was laudanum, 'as confirmed by people returning from the East, and by every Surgeon who goes there'. He also recommended red wine as 'very usefull and Phisicall for men sicke of ye ffux'; in 1627 the Company provided three hogsheads for their ships. For high fever, he advised reasonable purging and bleeding, but if there was no improvement, 'the body being open, then in the name of God give him a dose of Laudanum.'

In general, he warned that:

> over purging, bleeding, and much thin diet will be very dangerous at sea, and will surely turn your patient in to the Scurvy.

Woodall was well acquainted with scurvy.[5] He recognized that it was not only the most formidable of the diseases at sea but that it played a part in all the other diseases of sailors: 'I suppose if Seamen may be preserved from that disease, few other diseases would indanger them.' He gave explicit instructions for preventing and treating scurvy, recommending fresh fruit juice, orange, lime, or lemon (the best). As much of this as possible was to be carried from home, with a fresh supply to be taken on board at every landing, particularly in the Indies, as this was even more effective than that brought from home.

Surgeons on the early Company voyages took sixteenth century European medicine with them. This had features in common with Indian Medicine (p.13). Galen was still the dominant authority but this was changing as chemical drugs replaced herbals. His faulty anatomy, based mostly on animals, was being corrected by human dissections. His theory of the circulation of the blood – that the blood passed through pores in the heart – was disproved by William Harvey in 1628. Surgeons were finding that 'coction' (suppuration) was not essential for the healing of wounds (p.23).

The current diseases in Europe were plague, syphilis (for which mercury was being used instead of herbal mixtures), scurvy, smallpox, measles and other infectious diseases. 'Ague' (malaria) was common. Leprosy had almost completely disappeared. But medicine was concerned more with 'the condition of the sick man' and the balance of his humours than with specific diseases.

Witchcraft and sorcery had always been closely related to medical practice. During the sixteenth century the fear of witchcraft was fading, and punishments had become less severe. In the villages it was recognized that the 'wise' women did no harm and were often more helpful and cheaper than the doctors. The idea of demonic possession as the cause of mental illness was fading. But there was still a widespread belief in the supernatural and in the importance of astrological events in human affairs.

All medical practitioners were in conflict with the much larger number of quacks. The itinerant 'surgeon' would offer treatment that might be regarded as too hazardous by the qualified surgeon, using techniques handed down in his family for the treatment of conditions such as hernia, stone in the bladder and cataract. There was always a high complication rate, and these operations were only gradually brought into the main stream of practice.

The qualified surgeon, even when certificated by the Barbers' Company, was still of a lower social order than a physician with his university education. But the status of surgeons had been steadily rising throughout the sixteenth century. Knowledge of human anatomy had greatly improved as Galen's errors were corrected. New surgical expertise was being spread by books printed in the vernaculars which allowed men with no classical education to study the work of surgeons in different countries. The increasing use of gunpowder had changed the nature of wounds, and the techniques needed for their treatment created a demand for more trained surgeons. The doctrine that 'coction' (suppuration) was necessary for the healing of wounds had meant that surgeons were interfering with the natural healing process by filling wounds with salves and tampons to keep them open and promote the formation of pus. A wound inflicted by gunpowder was thought to be poisoned, and surgeons tried to destroy the poison by cautery or boiling oil. Paracelsus was one of the first to recognize that this apparent poisoning was the result of the scorching of the skin round the wound; he recommended simple cooling dressings. In the middle of the sixteenth century, Ambroise Paré, from his extensive experience as an army surgeon, had changed to a very gentle regime. His writings in the vernacular, and his great influence, meant that this new principle was generally adopted. It was the one recommended by Woodall.

Blood-letting was widely used for many different diseases, but no physician would soil his hands by such intimate contact with a patient; if he thought bleeding was necessary he would always call in a surgeon. Another very lucrative service provided by surgeons was the treatment of venereal disease. Syphilis was spreading rapidly; half the patients in St. Bartholomew's Hospital at any one time had the 'pox'. These calls on the surgeon's skill brought him greatly increased practice, adding to his income and status.[6]

The first Company surgeons had surgical texts in English for European diseases, and they had some idea of what to expect on the voyage, but little of what they would find on reaching India. There were many misconceptions:

People imagine that vast Country is all Gold, Silver, Pearls,

Diamonds and other precious Stones, but when a Man is in
the country, he soon finds much otherwise.

Poor men could be induced to sign on for the early voyages by unscrupulous agents who 'put a hammer into their hands to knock the diamonds out of the rocks they shall meet with'. The writings of merchants, travellers and missionaries were beginning to give more accurate accounts, although these contained very little medical detail, and this was often inaccurate, based on hearsay and local legend.

No specific works by Europeans on medicine in India were known before the second half of the sixteenth century. The first, by Garcia da Orta (1501-68), was published in Portuguese in Goa in 1563 and translated into Latin in 1567. Da Orta had reached India from Portugal in 1534 as physician to the Viceroy in Goa. He had a busy practice, not only the Portuguese but also many of the local rulers and noblemen. When called into consultation with the local physicians he always tried to learn from them. His experiences, describing the interaction of European and Indian medicine, were similar to those of the English in India in the early seventeenth century.

But his writings were in Latin, and so probably unintelligible to most of the Company surgeons.[7] He compared the European with the Indian methods of treatment and with those of the classical Arab physicians, finding that Avicenna had copied the Indians. He was critical of the Indians' lack of knowledge of anatomy, but he accepted that, guided by their pulse-lore, they gave satisfactory remedies to relieve suffering, and he acknowledged how much he had learned from them. There was clearly a ready exchange of medical ideas. The Portuguese doctors and druggists copied some of the Indian prescriptions, and the Indians learned to use European medicines. Da Orta made extensive studies of local plants and drugs. Many of them were already familiar, but if he was uncertain of the action of a drug he would take the advice of the brahmins. He recognized that treatment should be modified according to the constitution of the patient, especially in fevers. The Indians starved their patients for 10-15 days, giving them only fluids. This might be suitable for Hindus 'who eat nothing with blood', but he preferred to bleed and purge the more plethoric Europeans, and follow this with nourishing food.

Many of the local diseases were familiar to him, but cholera was much more severe than anything he had seen in Europe. Based on his experience of the epidemic in Goa in 1543, he gave the first description of what became known as Asiatic cholera:[8]

The victims died in a day or a day and a night. The mortality was so great that the bells would toll all day, and the Governor had to forbid them, so as not to frighten the people.

The Indian method of treatment was rice-water (with pepper and cummin) only to drink, cauterization of the soles of the feet, and binding the patient with strong bands to counteract the cramps. Da Orta did not believe in starvation, which was the mainstay of the Hindu treatment for most diseases. He recommended a small, but good, diet of best chicken eaten between slices of quince, after the patient had been cleansed with purges and clysters (enemas), but he cauterized the feet as the Indians did. He put his greatest faith in bezoar,[9] and claimed to have cured many patients in this way including the Bishop of Malacca.

Since Portuguese physicians were scarce in Goa, the Portuguese turned to the local practitioners, preferring them to their countrymen because of the Indians' greater knowledge of local diseases. The Indian doctors were credited with many cures, using their traditional remedies. They acquired great prestige, and were granted the special privilege of having an umbrella carried over them,

> like the Portingales which no other heathen doe, but Ambassadors, or some rich Merchants. These phisitions doe not onely cure there owne nations, but the Portingales also, for the Viceroy himselfe, the Archbishop, and all the Monkes and Friers doe put more trust in them, than in their own countriemen.

This favourable opinion began to change early in the seventeenth century. Portuguese physicians denounced Ayurvedic practitioners as mere faith healers, and they were prohibited from practice until they had taken an examination.

The Portuguese built the first hospital for Europeans in India in Goa. By the end of the sixteenth century it was being run by the Jesuits, with day-to-day care by Indians. A detailed account was given by Pyrard de Laval, a French sailor, who was captured by the Portuguese in 1607, and, when he fell ill, was taken there for three weeks for treatment. He was full of praise for the hospital, although he was generally contemptuous of the Portuguese. The hospital held up to fifteen hundred patients – Portuguese soldiers and other Christian Europeans. Although treatment was carried out skilfully there was a high mortality: 'every yeare there entered 500 live men, and never come forth till they are dead.' Among their diseases the most common were those which they call Mordexin [cholera], which kills immediately, burning feavers, and bloody fluxes [dysentery], against which they have no remedy but bleeding, which they resort to continually, and so long as the slightest feaver is present. The idolater Indians use not bleeding at all. The Plague is not known in the Indies; but, to make amends, they have the Pox, which destroys every year a great number ... it is no mark of shame there, nor any disgrace to have had it several times: they even make a boast of it. They cure it without sweating, with China root. This malady prevails only among the Christians.

The first book on tropical diseases in English was by George Wateson (1598), based on his experiences as a prisoner in Spain, but this reflected Spanish practice in the West Indies. Many of the treatments involved the use of tobacco, which the Spaniards had learned from the Amerindians. Wateson reminded the reader that more men are killed by sickness than by their enemies.

The work of the most distinguished Dutch physician in the East in the seventeenth century, Jacobus Bontius (1592-1631), was not translated into English until 1769. But two books by the Dutchman, Jan Huyghen van Linschoten, translated into English in 1598, were important sources of information. Born in Haarlem in 1563, Linschoten went to India with the Portuguese in 1583 on the staff of the Archbishop of Goa. After his return home he published his navigational experiences in 1595. Ships' captains on the early English expeditions relied on his detailed instructions for navigation through difficult channels and sandbanks. His second book (1596) was a general account of his experiences in India, the customs of its different races and classes, its flora and fauna, and the diseases that he encountered; the commonest of these were 'mordexin', 'the bloody Flixe' and 'continuall fevers'. They all carried a high mortality. He warned that the drugs sold by the brahmins were often dirty and 'full of garbish'.

Linschoten also described the deficiencies of the Portuguese, their defeats by the local inhabitants, their poor seamanship, and the degenerate breed that they were producing by their policy of encouraging mixed marriages. It was clear that they would not be such formidable opponents as their reputation in the East might have suggested, and that their colonial empire was 'rotten, and ripe for conquest'.

Notes

1 A charter was essential for a regulated company; without it all trades and crafts were illegal.

2 The United Company of Barbers and Surgeons had been formed in 1540 with the power of licensing surgeons, and the duty of providing surgeons for the Navy. Approved candidates were apprenticed to practising surgeons.

3 Surgeons were forbidden to prescribe medicines – only a member of the College of Physicians of London was qualified for this.

4 This reached its fourth edition in 1655. Copies of the first edition are now very rare; perhaps the young surgeons wore them out with over-use. After the first edition Woodall added a section on plague for which he used his own antidote, *aurum vitae*, containing gold.

5 Due to deficiency of vitamin C.
Woodall's advice was 150 years before James Lind's experiments (p.114), and 200 years before the supply of fresh juice became official policy in the Navy.

6 'Experience teaching us every day, that one Pocky Whore brings the Surgeon more Grist in, than a thousand *French* cannon. Next to Whores, Punch is his best Friend, that being an approv'd fomenter of Blood and Wounds, which brings him in many more Crown-pieces, than ever he had from his Father.'

7 One of the few able to study da Orta was Richard Surflet who took the book on the second Company voyage (1604). He had been educated at Cambridge, and was in holy orders and licensed to practise physic. He was employed by the Company as chaplain and surgeon. He proved to be an incompetent surgeon, much disliked by the sailors. He died of scurvy on the homeward voyage.

8 Da Orta used the terms *morxi* or *mordexi* (from the Mahratti 'collapsed'), later corrupted by the French to *mort-de-chien* (a 'dog's death'), which was widely adopted by later traders.

9 Bezoar – a soft stone found in the stomach of various animals (p.242).

Chapter Four
The early voyages (1601-23)

The first English expedition of four ships and a pinnace of provisions left London on 13 February 1601 under the command of Captain James Lancaster in his flagship, *Red Dragon*, with a crew of 200 men and a surgeon. They reached Achin (Sumatra) on 5 June 1602. Here they found the price of pepper very high, and there was little demand for the heavy cloth that they had brought. Lancaster's solution was to capture a passing Portuguese galleon and use part of her huge cargo for barter. A factory (trading post) was set up at Bantam (Java) in December 1602. *Red Dragon* set out for home on 20 February 1603, reaching London in September 1603 loaded with pepper and other spices. Out of the combined crews of 460 men, 182 had died. The second expedition, under Henry Middleton, left in March 1604, reaching Bantam on 22 December, and returned in May 1606. These two expeditions showed a profit of 95 per cent.

The Dutch were already established in the East Indies. From their arrival in 1596 they had adopted a very aggressive policy, and had soon abolished local Arab, Indian and Chinese competition, and instituted forced labour. They were also destructive – capturing and laying waste spice-producing land, in order to keep the prices up. They were hated for their brutal behaviour and drunkenness. When the Chinese on Formosa captured fourteen Dutchmen,

> remembering how cruel the Hollanders had been to their Nation ... they put out one eye of each, cut off their Noses, Ears, and one Hand, and so sent them back ... to tell ... that the Dutch had taught them that kind of mercy.

The soldiers and junior servants of the two trading Companies were continually quarrelling, but the seniors of both nations at first treated each other with courtesy. The Dutch were notably kind to the survivors of Middleton's expedition when they reached Bantam in December 1604 with only 50 healthy men.

The third English expedition sailed in 1607. William Hawkins, with one ship, was detached to set up the first English factory in India, in 1608, at Surat, the most important port of the Mogul Empire and the port of embarcation of the pilgrims for Mecca. Hawkins, who was a hard drinker, got on well with the Emperor Jahangir[1] at his Court in Agra but found it impossible to make any firm trading agreement. The two ships of the fourth expedition were lost. By 1610 the Company had sent out 17 ships, and the Dutch 60 ships.

On the seventh voyage (1611-15 under Peter Floris) trading was started in the Bay of Bengal, with a profit of 218 per cent. This was encroaching on the favourite sites of the Dutch, and caused friction which eventually led to open war. By 1611 the English still had only a small settlement at Bantam, but there was now agreement with Jahangir to trade at Surat and three other places around the Gulf of Cambay. Trading was started with Persia, and John Saris led the first English expedition to Japan in 1613. Trading with the mainland of India brought the English into conflict with the Portuguese, who had built up their empire by ruthless conquest, and whose forceful trading was accompanied by fierce missionary zeal and the terrors of the Inquisition. In order to make up their small numbers, their men were encouraged to marry local women, particularly those who had been converted, but their offspring were often of poor quality. Their power was already fading, and their prestige was further lowered by defeats at sea by the smaller ships of the tenth English expedition under Thomas Best (1612-14). These battles took place close enough to the shore for the humiliation of the Portuguese to be witnessed by Indians on land. The news spread widely, and improved the prospects of the English for trading in Western India.

The Indians favoured the English because, unlike the Portuguese and the Dutch, they had, at first, no territorial ambitions and they were tolerant of their religions. But Jesuits (who had arrived in Goa in 1542) were in Agra, and were petitioning the Emperor against the English. The merchants in Surat appealed to James I for support.

Sir Thomas Roe was sent out with the full panoply of an Ambassador, sailing on 4 March 1615 in a fleet of four ships, reaching India on 26 September. He then had a 600-mile journey to reach the Mogul Court on 23 December. He suffered recurrent bouts of fever, and arrived so weak that he was unable to attend the *durbar* (the Emperor's daily meeting at the Court) until 20 January:

> Since my arrival in this country, I have had but one month of health and that mingled with relapses, and am now your poor servant scarce a crow's dinner.

As a nobleman he was courteously received, but the presents that he brought – lavish by European standards – were thought to be hardly worthy as from one king to another. The Emperor was delighted with the state coach, but its lining of red cloth was thought to be more suitable for covering elephants, and was replaced by richer material; the iron nails were replaced by gold. After prolonged negotiations Roe obtained a *firman* (permit) which allowed further factories to be set up.

In 1620 the Portuguese were again defeated at sea, but the Dutch now began to attack the English in the East Indies for interfering with their trade. In February 1623 they extracted 'confessions' under torture from the servants of the sixteen men in the English factory at Amboyna. Trumped-up charges of plotting to overthrow the Dutch Governor were brought. The English were arrested, tortured, and, all except two, executed on 23 February – the 'Massacre at Amboyna'. The English then abandoned their factories in the East Indies to concentrate on the mainland of India with their headquarters at Surat.

Over the first twelve voyages the Company's profit was 138 per cent. By 1621 2,500 seamen were employed. Their medical problems started on the voyage. Throughout the sixteenth century larger ships were being built to cope with longer voyages. Improved navigation allowed the ships to stand out to sea and avoid the hazards of coastal waters. The risk of the crew picking up infection at every landing place was reduced, but the likelihood of epidemics spreading in the crowded conditions on board was increased, and in any ship that had been at sea for two-three months, or longer with storms and contrary winds, without fresh provisions, scurvy was almost inevitable.

The outward voyage via the Cape of Good Hope took up to six months and sometimes longer. The ships sailed at the end of winter, usually January or February, in order to round the Cape in time to catch the south-west monsoon that would take them on to the west coast of India (p. 1). The Cape was the half-way mark, and it was an important staging post for re-victualling and allowing sickly crews some time on land. It was the custom to sing the *Te Deum* when safely round, for there was then 'some assurance of compleating the Voyage, whereof the Cape makes one half.'

An intermediate landing at St. Helena was favoured by the English, as it had been stocked by the Portuguese with animals and fruit, and there was plenty of good water. Sick men could be left there, living in tents. The animals were so plentiful that they could be killed with sticks and stones, and fish could be caught with crooked nails. The ships would then pick the men up on the way back the following year. On the way home from the Cape, it was vital to call there. Once past, it was impossible to turn back because of the south-east wind, and the last leg of the voyage was then

> the greatest miserie in ye world ... for those ships that miss it being in an ill state, ready to be eaten up with the Scurvy.

Lack of fresh food or fruit meant that scurvy was inevitable on any long voyage. It was 'the plague of the sea, and the spoyle of mariners'. Many of the ordinary seamen, recruited from the lowest classes, were already unhealthy, worse in times of poor harvests, bringing disease with them on board. In addition, they were probably 'pre-scorbutic'[2] as a result of a deficient diet through the winter.

The dramatic effects of scurvy – blotched ulcerated limbs, rotting gums with teeth falling out, men too weak to crawl even under threat of punishment, and often dying suddenly – with no known cure, were often recorded.

> Never mine eyes such dreary sight beheld,
> Ghastly the mouth and gums enormous swell'd.
> And instant, putrid like a dead man's wound,
> Poisoned with foetid steams the air around,
> No sage physician's ever-watchful zeal,
> No skilful surgeon's gentle hand to heal
> Were found: each dreary mournful hour we gave
> Some brave companion to a foreign grave.[3]

This was 'sea' scurvy. But there had always been a similar, although less severe, disorder on land – a little lassitude, blotching and scaly eruptions on the skin, and spongy bleeding gums. 'Land' scurvy had been noted since Roman times, particularly among the very poor and in prisons and sieges, most marked in the winter and improving in the spring. Until the middle of the seventeenth century they were thought to be separate diseases.[4] The winter diet of most people, rich and poor, in England in the sixteenth century contained very little vitamin C, and the levels of this would have been at their lowest at the end of the winter. There were many recommended remedies for making loose teeth firm and 'purifying the blood' in the spring, mostly fresh green-stuff, particularly scurvy-grass (spoon-wort, *Cochlearia officinalis*). It was recognized that boiling these remedies would destroy their efficacy, and that it was impossible to preserve them at sea.

As all the early voyages set out in the middle of winter, it is probable that many or most of the crew, and even some of the officers and merchants, were already in a pre-scorbutic state before the start of the voyage. All ships' captains expected scurvy to break out once the ship had been at sea for more than two months.[5] By the time they reached the Cape – on a 'good' voyage in three months – there might already be widespread disease. If the ship was becalmed or delayed by storms, or blown round the Cape without being able to land, the ship could be paralysed by the number of casualties, with not enough fit men to set the sails or man the guns. The mortality was high, and those who survived ran a greatly increased risk of intercurrent disease, particularly dysentery, either at sea or on landing.

The feature of scurvy that was most often noted was the general weakness and lethargy. Even under threat of severe punishment the men had not the strength to work the ship. 'Idleness' was at first thought to be one of the causes of scurvy, to be treated by the bosun's cane:

> this small stick of his, has wonderful Vertues in it, and seems little inferior to the Rod of Moses, of miraculous Memory; it has cur'd more of the Scurvy, than the Doctor, and made many a poor Cripple take up his bed and walk.

Minor wounds would not heal, and old wounds that had been healed for twenty years or more would break open. This was seen particularly in prisoners and men under punishment where the abrasions from chafing of the fetters quickly turned to gangrene. Standard punishments had to be modified or abandoned.

The high death rate in the closed community of a ship lowered the spirits of the survivors:

> The Loss of a Man ought to be taken notice of in a Nation, or in a City, when there are thousands still left, how much more considerable is such a Loss to us, who have so few in this our Wooden World.

With fewer hands, they were under even greater strain in working the ship. The sailors, soaked, overworked and underfed, were always more affected than their officers and the merchants who had private means and access to extra supplies in the stores.

There was continued speculation about possible positive causes,[6] of which the commonest was excess salt – salt meat in the diet and salt in the sea air. The Dutch, from the middle of the sixteenth century, were the first to realize the benefits of fresh fruit. Attempts were made to preserve the virtue of the fresh juice, but it was soon found that this was destroyed by boiling.[7] There was some success from adding rum or other spirits (p. 114).

The first Company captain to use lemon juice was James Lancaster, taking bottles of it on the first voyage (1601). When they reached Table Bay, his ship was the only one of the four with a relatively fit and efficient crew. In the other ships the sickness rate was so high that the merchants had to take their turn at the helm and even 'go into the top' to trim the sails 'as the common mariners did'. Most of the sick recovered after some time on land, but already 105 men had died out of 460. On the onward voyage Lancaster advised the ships to put into land to pick up fresh oranges and lemons, but in spite of this a further 77 had died by the time the fleet got home.

Middleton, on the second voyage (1604), took some lemon juice, but it was not enough to last them to Table Bay. As they passed the Line, there were many with scurvy and dysentery. Middleton wanted to press on round the Cape, but the sick men

> cryed out most lamentebly, at least eighty in the ship, not one able to helpe the other. The Generall looking out of his cabin doors, where did attend a swarme of lame and weake, diseased cripples, graunted their requests.

They reached Bantam with only fifty healthy men in the four ships, and Middleton himself 'very sickely and weake'. Some of the sick died soon after arrival, and even some of those who arrived in reasonable health died.

> Bantam is not a place to recover men that are sicke, but rather to kill men that come thither in health.

On subsequent voyages 'lemon water' was included in the victualling lists, but supplies often ran out or became ineffective, and ships were unable to land for fresh supplies. The sickness rate remained high.

John Woodall drew together the experiences of the early voyages in his instructions to young Company surgeons in 1617 (p.20). He thought that the salt diet was the main cause and he knew that the remedies on land could not be preserved at sea. The best treatment was fruit juice. Lemon was the best of all, but it should be kept for the men, and not wasted by using it as a sauce for the officers' meat. He advised that

> the Chirurgion or his mate must not faile to perswade the Governour or Purser in all places where they touch in the Indies and may have it, to provide themselves of juice of Oranges, limes or lemons, and at Banthame of Tamarinds.

Once the fresh fruit had run out, all other remedies at sea were useless, and the only hope was to get the men on shore as soon as possible.

After scurvy the commonest disease was the 'flux', either *de novo* or as a complication of scurvy. On Middleton's voyage two or three men died from this every day, including the ship's cook and the baker.

The 'callenture' (possibly heatstroke) was a disease peculiar to ships in the tropics, which could occur like an epidemic. The victims had a high fever, causing them to believe 'the spacious sea and waves therein to be great fields full of haycocks', into which they would joyfully try to throw themselves unless restrained. It was sometimes impossible to rescue them as the ship could not be turned in time. Attempts would be made to revive a drowned man by cutting the end off a knife-sheath, thrusting it into his fundament and 'blowing until weary, and then get others to continue' – occasionally successful. Sometimes tobacco smoke was blown in.

A major factor in the high mortality on long voyages was overcrowding. The ships were sent out with more men than for a coastal voyage to compensate for the expected deaths, and to ensure that there were enough men to bring the ships home. This led to the problem of feeding such numbers, and ensured the rapid spread of infectious diseases. The foul atmosphere below decks was made worse in bad weather when hatches had to be closed to prevent flooding. In a storm everything would get soaked so that if the 'Seamen lay Cloaths by for 24 hours, they become all full of little Maggots'. Soldiers and other passengers, unused to these conditions and the dietary restrictions of a long voyage, were particularly vulnerable. The English were more careful about overcrowding than the Dutch and the Portuguese whose grossly overmanned ships might lose half their numbers on the outward voyage. But it still took time and repeated pleas from the surgeons for the Company to appreciate the false economy of overmanning, and that it would be cheaper to provide proper care for smaller numbers.

The ships were sometimes short of men because of impressment for the Navy. Naval ships could hail a merchantman and press as many fit men as they needed. The men would feign illness or deformity to escape, but their ships might have to anchor or turn back for lack of men. At home, replacements could be found. In the East, men were always hired locally to help load and unload, but they might also be needed to make up the crews for the homeward voyage. These Indian sailors (lascars), accustomed to short coastal voyages, were often unsuited to long ocean voyages. They were repatriated as soon as possible on the next Company voyage. While waiting for a ship they were lodged in London, often in squalid conditions so that they were a source of infection when they came on board.

Fire was a constant hazard and burns were common, not only in sea-battles where fire-ships and incendiary missiles were used but also from carelessness when handling flints, matches and candles, and from the cooks' fires, and powder explosions. The fire-risk was made greater by the whole ship being 'all pitchy and tarry' and the large quantities of spirits commonly carried (Indian arrack burned even more fiercely than European brandy), and by inflammable cargoes of spices and gums. Once a fire had started it was difficult to stop it spreading. The ceremonial firing of cannon as a mark of respect or in celebration could lead to injuries and deaths – a gunner in 1608 'shooting a peace in welcome blew awaye an arme, whereof he dyed'.

Disease was always the major cause of death at sea. Thomas Best kept notes of the casualties on the tenth voyage (1612-14). Out of a total of 220 men in two ships, 99 died of illness (most of these while the ships were in the East Indies), 2 in accidents, and 3 had been killed in battles with the Portuguese.

All the Company's ships were armed, and prepared to fight to defend themselves, or to attack their rivals in trade. Ships of under 500 tons with a crew of 90 carried 30 guns. There were no naval convoys until the late eighteenth century, and even then naval protection might not extend further than the Channel or St. Helena. Pirates of various nations were common off the Malabar (west) Coast. They were easily beaten off by the Company's ships but they often attacked smaller coastal vessels:

> nor is the voyage safe on account of the Malabars ... these People take poor Passengers, and lest they should have swallow'd their Gold, tho' they have no need of it, give them a Potion, which makes them Digest all they have in their Bodies, which done, they search the stinking Excrements to find the precious Metal.

Everybody was allocated duties in case of battle. Portuguese ships always carried large numbers of soldiers who were brave but useless until the ships got to close quarters. This was often prevented by the superior seamanship and gunnery of the English. But Nicholas Downton (captain of the 1614-15 voyage) described the disadvantages under which his men were fighting:

> Before my people came to fight they are first tired or halfe spent with the labour of the ship, as heaving at capstains and getting up our anchors, setting of sailes and other labours, which greatly quells their courage, making them in hot countreys both weary and faint, and then of necessitie must become souldiours; whereas the Viceroy his souldiours come fresh to fight, being troubled with no labour which is done by slaves and inferiour sea-people ... if the Viceroy loose many men in his ships he may be supplyed againe out of his fresh supplyes to be fetcht from their nearest townes by their frigates; whereas we could not have one man supplyed, how many soever we should have slaine or disabled.

Discipline on board was strict. Instructions from the Directors forbade blaspheming or swearing; penalties ranged from 'three blows' to 24 hours in the bilboes (on bread and water, chained by the ankle to a bar in the hold). There was to be no dicing or playing at cards. Challenges to a duel or duelling were punished with forty lashes and a spell in the bilboes. Drunkenness at sea led to disorder, and was always severely punished.

Chaplains were first appointed to the ships on the second voyage (1604); they often had some medical knowledge. Every member of the crew had to attend divine service every morning and evening. Left to themselves, the sailors were less devout. In the worst storms there was 'no impression on the sailors to prayer', and they only swore the louder; it needed a battle at sea against extreme odds. In a shipwreck there was always a lot of cursing, but after the ship was wrecked they would take to the boats 'singing of psalmes to the praise of God'.

Attempts were made to keep the ship clean and sweet at all times. The ship's ports were opened whenever possible to air the ship, and the foul air below deck was cleared by burning damp gunpowder or juniper, or spraying with vinegar. The cooks had to keep their pots clean, especially the steeptubs (for soaking salt meat before cooking); the penalty for failure was 24 hours in the bilboes. The homeward voyage was often cleaner. There were fewer men, the survivors were richer and could provide their own necessities, and the ship was sweet with spices.

The Directors' instructions included the care of the sick. They were to be kept clean and well fed, and the surgeons were to do their best for them. Every ship was expected to carry a surgeon and a mate but there were many casualties among them. When a surgeon was available, the mate's duties were relatively simple: 'boiling gruel, barley-water fomentations, washing rollers, making lint, spreading plaisters, and fitting the dresses ... and emptying the buckets they went to stool in'. He was also expected to pull teeth and barber the ship's company. Full surgeons might be only on the larger ships. The smaller ships would have only a mate, who might have 'scarce skill enough to bleed a man'. There were complaints that they neglected the sailors, while giving their time to the officers and passengers who were, in any case, likely to be healthier than the men because of their better diet and living conditions:

> ... careless of a poor man in his sickness ... their common phrase being to come to him and take him by the hand when they hear that he hath been sick two or three days and feeling his pulses when he is half dead, asking him when he was at stool and how he feels himself, and how he has slept, and then giving him some of their medicines upon the point of a

knife, which doeth as much good to him as a blow upon the pate with a stick.

But many of the surgeons were highly commended and valuable members of the ship's company. Practice at sea could be hard on them – 'fractured limbs are unhappy cases to manage in a gale'. They worked in cramped conditions, and in a battle

> when I was amputating the limb of one of our wounded seamen, the very shaking of the lower gun-deck just over head, is of itself sufficient to incommode a surgeon.

On long voyages all food had to be dried or salted but even this might not prevent deterioration. Drying meant that the food had to be soaked, and this used up precious supplies of water. The staple diet was dry biscuit with salt beef or pork boiled in salt water; this was thought to be the cause of the bloody flux which was so common in sailors. The ships only loaded the correct amount of food for the estimated length of the voyage. If this was prolonged by storms, the men had to go short or spend part of their wages on food. The officers and merchants had separate stores and always fared better. Every ship carried livestock which used up water and fouled the ship with droppings. Gardens were set up on deck to provide fresh vegetables. Most of this fresh food was reserved for the officers and merchants. In a storm it might all be washed overboard. When the ship was in danger all cargo on deck might have to be jettisoned including the water casks.

Stocks were replenished at every port. If the ship could call at Ascension the turtles there would provide good fresh meat. But in the tropics, even when fresh meat could be obtained 'the great difficulty is to salt it, for before it can take salt it will stink'. Life at sea was often dependent on catching fish; dolphins always made a good meal. One crew had the melancholy experience of catching a shark, and finding inside it the body of their sergeant lost overboard a short while before, and 'none could find in their Heart to Eat of the Fish'. On shorter voyages the provisions were more lavish. For the nineteen days of a passage from Persia to Surat in April 1636 the Captain's table was

> well furnished with Fowls, Mutton, and other fresh meat, but above all things, with excellent good Sack, English Beer, French Wines, Arak, and other refreshments.

The rations for the crew were sack and biscuit for breakfast, and two main meals of beef or wheat and honey on alternate days alternating with rice and honey or oatmeal, with pork or beef occasionally.

The supply and preservation of water was a major problem. Drinking water was carried on deck in oak casks in which sulphur had been burned to kill the worms. The casks were filled at every opportunity, but the water quickly deteriorated. In the tropics, fresh rainwater became full of small worms in less than four hours. The crew were used to drinking foul water. If it became particularly foul it was treated by dropping in a red-hot cannonball. Even such murky fluid was often in short supply. Strict rationing was then enforced although the diet might only be dry biscuit and salt beef boiled in salt water. Thames water had the reputation of staying fresher than any other and it was always kept till last. It might have an oily scum (which was highly inflammable) when the cask was opened, but 'let it stand unbunged on the Deck twenty four hours, it recovers its goodness'. Opening the casks was always hazardous:

> the Coopers affirm they are as cautious to strike
> with their Adds on the Cask for fear it taking fire,
> as of Brandy itself.

Attempts were made to obtain fresh water by distilling from sea-water. The best method had to be abandoned because it used up too much firewood, and the early results were so unpalatable that the men would not drink it.

With the shortage of water, alcohol was in even greater demand than usual. Large quantities were always carried. There was a regular ration which might be increased in times of stress and hardship – 'to everye man 1 pynt of wyne for laboring in getting the ship of the rocks.' It was also valued for its medicinal properties; red wine was particularly recommended for the flux. There were frequent calls by the surgeons for more supplies for their patients.

The ships usually carried enough salt meat and biscuit for the whole voyage, but it was essential to land if supplies of water or wood ran out or if there were too many sick men. The quickest way to cure a sailor of scurvy was to put him on shore.

But there were hazards on land. In any developed port there were always venereal diseases, and after any period of shore leave some of the crew would be 'clapt and poxt'. In the tropics, even to anchor in harbour was dangerous:

> After the rain there came a sweet smell from shore, as if new-
> cut herbs or hay, which did prove very ominous, for some of

our men fell sick that very night; and that week we had one hundred at least down at once.

On landing in search of water, there were warnings not to stray too far from the coast and to show good behaviour to the local inhabitants. But lives were lost in fights with hostile natives. The search often took up a great deal of time and labour, and was sometimes fruitless. Even if a fresh spring was found, transporting the casks was 'a laboure beyond measure' for the exhausted crew. It was especially dangerous to spend the night on shore, when 'agues' would certainly follow. Prudent captains learned to ensure that all the crew were back on board before dark and the ship anchored well away from the land and its pestilential 'miasma'.

The survivors of the hardships and dangers of a voyage that might have lasted six months or more then had to face the largely unknown conditions in India as they landed at Surat, the first English settlement on the mainland.

Notes

1 Jahangir had succeeded his father, Akbar, in 1605. Akbar, who ruled from 1556, was the grandson of Babur, founder of the Mogul Empire (1526). Jahangir was addicted to opium and alcohol.

2 A mild degree of vitamin C deficiency, not fully recognized until the 1920s.

3 Garcia da Orta's contemporary, Camoëns, describing Vasco da Gama's crew (1497-8) as they reached the east coast of Africa.

4 There were no accounts of scurvy in India at this time. It was not realized until the nineteenth century that scurvy was common in some of the poorer villages, particularly in the winter, and that outbreaks could occur in Indian troops (p.192).

5 Vitamin C cannot be stored in the body – a daily intake is necessary for health.

6 The idea that a disease could be due to the absence of something did not come until the early twentieth century when the relation between vitamins and 'deficiency diseases' was first being discussed.

7 It was not until the early nineteenth century that canning was developed and shown to be an effective preservative.

Chapter Five
Arrival in India

By the time the English arrived in the early seventeenth century India had been under Muslim rule for four hundred years. After the Emperor Akbar (reigned 1556-1605), his son, Jahangir (reigned 1605-27), continued the policy of toleration of Hindus. The vast mass of the people were left in peace, as long as they paid their taxes. But the collection of taxes was left in the hands of local Hindu rulers who often treated the people harshly. The Mogul Court at Agra was the most magnificent in the world, and there were a few very rich men, but India was, in general, a poor country. There was no margin for a bad harvest and the resulting famine. The population had been growing relatively rapidly from the end of the fifteenth century, and this increased the frequency and severity of famine.

The English, at first, found it difficult to distinguish the different races in India, and divided them broadly into 'Moors' (Muslims) and 'Heathens' (Hindus). Landing on the west coast where the Jains[1] predominated, they thought that their extreme non-violence, their concern for all living things, and their animal 'hospitals' (p. 55) were the pattern all over India. They came to prefer the Muslims as the rulers who could further their trading interests. It took them some time to realize that Muslims lumped all Europeans and Hindus together as heathen worshippers of idols, and that brahmins[2] regarded Europeans and Muslims as *farangis*,[3] considering them to be spiritually little better than the lowest estate.

The English soon found that the banyans[4] were more subtle and financially skilled than the Muslims, and they chose them as their brokers. But they were handicapped by not knowing any local language, and they did not take the trouble to learn one.[5] Communication was in pidgin Portuguese, used by traders all over the East. The alternative was an interpreter, but this all led to misunderstandings and complaints of fraud. The first opinions of the English about Indians were based on their dealings with banyans. They noted their religious exercises and care for animals,

> but yet for all this lousie scruple, they stick not at cozenage by false weights, measures and coyne, nor at usury and lies.

The Company always urged honest behaviour as the surest way to get goodwill to promote trading – 'righteousness is at the root of our prosperity.'

But some of the early recruits were of poor calibre, insolent and brutal, and were responsible for the low opinion that Indians developed for the English.[6] But the Indians had bitter memories of the Portuguese and were prepared to support the English against them. The Portuguese tried to persuade the local ruler to poison the well that the English used,

> but the Ethnike had more honestie, and put in quicke
> Tortoises, that it might appeare by their death if any venomous
> hand had beene there.

The senior officers of the Company were generally civil, and Indians learned to distinguish them from their riotous juniors. If they behaved peaceably they were safe with the Indians, 'amongst whom our nation hath found much good respect, and little affront or injury'.

As they started to move inland, the English found that the country was peaceful. There were officials with troops to keep the highways free from robbers. Contact with the people was mostly at the courts of the rulers where they were suppliants for protection for their poorly manned factories and for the *firman* (permit) to continue trading. They were anxious to show their respect and they were prepared to take off their boots and kneel with their heads to the ground. But anyone whom the Indians regarded as a nobleman would often be honoured for his refusal to conform. Sir Thomas Roe (p. 30) demanded a chair, and refused to bow to the Emperor. He was not given a chair but remained upright propped against a pillar, and he gained respect for this.

Contact with higher-caste Hindus was limited by their fear of pollution so that they were not able to eat at each other's tables. The habits of the Muslims were more congenial:

> the Moores drink wine and spirits liberally, but the Banians
> only drink water, and are fat and sleek from confectuaries of
> all sorts.

The monotheistic religion of Muslims was familiar as compared with the many Hindu gods. The concern of the Hindus for all forms of life was a barrier to the sporting habits of the English who were warned 'not to kill anything in the countries of the Rajas'. A merchant who shot a peacock was whipped until he died. But there were no such dangers in areas 'where the rulers are Muhammedans and permit sport to be free'.

The English contrasted the warlike behaviour of the Muslims with the peacefulness of the Hindus. But they marvelled at the strict caste rules which ensured that a Hindu would rather die of starvation than 'touch Christian meate'.[7] The wandering yogis and fakirs attracted wonder for their austerities, but more often excited scorn:

> in Patanaw I saw a dissembling prophet who made as though he slept, and many of the people came and touched his feet. They took him for a great man but sure he was a lazy lubber. I left him there sleeping. The people of these countries are much given to such prating and dissembling hypocrites.

The Company was, at first, noted for its piety; all its servants had to be Protestants. Chaplains were sent out with the early voyages. They were impressed with the religious freedom in India. They found much that appalled them in the religion of the Hindus, but they praised their good habits of prayer and abstemiousness with food and drink, particularly the ban on alcohol. They preached these virtues, and urged them on their dissolute compatriots.

Missionaries, at this time, were tolerated by the Company. They usually had some medical knowledge and this helped them to make contact with the people. They took the trouble to learn the local languages, and, as they were mostly remote from the towns, they were often the only medical advice available. Later, as the Company's political power increased, missionaries were banned from entering India for fear that they would unsettle the local population. By the nineteenth century the Company had become known as 'the ungodly Company'.

If the English came to admire some aspects of Hinduism, there were customs that they found abhorrent, particularly suttee[8] (burning widows). They thought, at first, that this was to deter lecherous women from poisoning their husbands in favour of their lovers, but they learned that it was a matter of honour. If the woman was prevented from burning on her husband's pyre, or her courage failed, her head was shaved, and she and her family were permanently disgraced. The Muslim rulers were generally opposed to the custom and tried to persuade the women not to conform. But if they were adamant, the Muslims and, later, the English, were reluctant to interfere with such an entrenched custom. Sometimes the horrified English tried to rescue the women – occasionally with a happy outcome. Job Charnock, founder of Calcutta, married the widow of a brahmin, whom he had rescued (p.78).

The English noted, and usually deplored, the open sexuality of the Hindus and the large number of aphrodisiacs in their pharmacopoeias. They recognized the classification of substances and drugs as 'hot' or 'cold', but 'in India this means that a drug is given either to promote or repress aphrodisia'. They were scornful of the need for such supports:

> by reason of the great Heat ... their Bodies being weaker than in cold Countries, and requiring a greater support for the Pleasures of Love.

They were living in an age of cruelty, but they repeatedly commented on the wanton cruelty of Indian rulers although they were often generous to the poor. One ruler, entertaining his English guests with the usual troupe of dancing girls, summoned a second troupe from the city. When they did not come at once, he had them brought before him and ordered their heads to be cut off in the presence of his guests. Seeing his guests' dismay, he laughed, saying that if he did not punish disobedience in this way he could never continue as ruler of the city. Punishment by the English was always harsh, but it was defined by law or custom so that the offender knew what to expect. The death-penalty by hanging was carried out with little delay after sentence had been passed. Mutineers were blown from the mouth of a gun – 'painless to the criminal and terrible to the beholder'. But Indian rulers devised grisly methods of punishment and long-drawn-out execution according to their mood at the time. The English recorded these in detail, expressing their horror, but they were unwilling to interfere as this might prejudice their trading activities.

In the sixteenth and early seventeenth centuries the English had the reputation in Europe of being rough and piratical. But they compared favourably in the East with the proud and bigoted 'Portugals' and the bullying 'Hollanders'. The Company, with its strong Puritan background, always tried to discipline its servants in good behaviour. All the trading companies had continual trouble over private trading by their employees which distracted them from their loyalty to the company, and reduced profits. The English Directors prohibited private trading, but salaries were so low that all their servants were involved in private trade. Instructions from London, even on the quickest voyages, took so long to get through that the men in India, faced with some crisis, had to take immediate decisions. They often found that, when the instructions did arrive, their masters at home had little experience of the problem, and their advice was impractical and better disobeyed.

The Company was always trying to economize and was anxious not to build up a large professional army. Their soldiers were as poorly paid as the rest of their servants, and Indian rulers tempted some of the best ones away. Europeans were always in demand to train Indian armies, particularly in artillery and engineering. They were either deliberately recruited, or, more commonly, had deserted in search of more favourable conditions where their duties were light and they were reputed to have 'great stipends and marry heathen women'. But those who wished to come back often found it hard to get away, as their new masters would not release them.

The Company's soldiers were often of poor quality, and generally despised by the merchants to whom they were subordinate. The Directors insisted that, at all times, the civilians should have authority over the soldiers, and

> when there was fighting to be done, the command was taken by factors and writers,[9] who were given commissions for the occasion.

At first there were relatively few troops, and the civilians, including the surgeons, were expected to know how to fight, and to be prepared to turn out at short notice whenever necessary.

No English women accompanied the early expeditions. Only in the latter part of the seventeenth century did the Company allow women to go out to India. The Portuguese had encouraged marriage between their soldiers and Indian women, and treated the offspring as Portuguese citizens, hoping in this way to increase the numbers of their nation in India. The Dutch allowed marriage with Indian women, but the women had to become Christian first. The English Company strongly disapproved of marriage to Indians, but, in spite of denunciations from the chaplains, many of their servants lived with local women. This taught them something of the customs of the country.[10] Many of these liaisons lasted long and faithfully. They were an important part of the generally peaceful relations in this early period between English and Indians, which would change towards the end of the seventeenth century as the military and political power of the Company increased.

There were many misunderstandings. The first Jesuit missionaries believed that they had discovered a nation of Catholics – Buddhist ritual has similarities to that of Rome. The Emperor Jahangir, one of whose titles was 'Conqueror of the World', was upset by the size of the world outside his empire when Sir Thomas Roe showed him the *Cosmography* of Mercator in 1615. But the first English traders were tolerated when it was seen that they were not trying to invade the country, although by defeating the Portuguese they had impressed the Indians with their fighting power. They had strict instructions from their masters at home to treat Indians with courtesy and honesty, and offences against Indians were severely punished. They were prepared to show proper deference to the local rulers and they made no attempt to interfere with Indian religions.

They adopted some of the local customs of dress and food, but this was mainly for comfort and to further their trading interests. They tended to keep together in their small communities for protection and to counter the feeling of loneliness among the vast numbers of Indians and the constant threat of death from overwhelming disease in the unaccustomed heat.

They were unprepared for the intense heat of the hot season which first hit them in the Persian Gulf where the heat was the most unbearable of anywhere in the East. The winds were so stifling that they could destroy men and animals. Even on the Carnatic (east coast of India), a place containing 5-10,000 inhabitants might lose four or five a day:

> many of the natives are in their travail suffocated and perish. And of Christians, a Dutchman, as hee was carried in his palankeene, and an Englishman walking but from the towne, little above an English mile dyed.
>
> The feebleness and languor both of body and mind, consequent upon excessive heat, may be considered a species of unremitting malady, which attacks all persons indiscriminately.

The pestilential air of the land was as dangerous as the heat and could attack the ships anchored in harbour – 'through strong pestilential feavers we lost most of our principal officers, including the surgeon.' The most profitable trading areas were often the worst. The Malabar (west) Coast of India was famous for pepper, and it might be

> very fruitfull, greene and pleasant to beholde, but it hath a very noysome and pestiferous ayre for such as are not borne in the countrie.

The East Indies were even more dangerous. The early English voyages went there because it was the centre for trade in all the richest goods from a wide area, but

> I do wish all our nation never to attempt the sendynge of our men ... for so contagious is there the ayre, and the water so evell, that is unpossible for a Christian to live.

Many of the men reached India in poor health from the rigours of the voyage. They were vulnerable to the new diseases that they were exposed to on land. From the first, the mortality was very high, even by contemporary European standards. But, apart from the numbers who died, it was the speed with which death occurred that confused and frightened the survivors. John Downes 'sitting att diner att noon, was dead at night'. Thomas Essington 'att noone eate his dinner ... dead at 5'; it was thought that he might have been bewitched. Sir Thomas Roe's chaplain, John Hall, died on 19 August 1616:

hee had been ill but 5 dayes, and that but easely. In the morning he had walked abroad, and lay downe in a Garden on the wett Earth, supposing him selfe in no danger. At noone hee eate with very good appetite. In two howers after he dyed.

With no experience of living and working in tropical conditions the English brought their regular habits with them. They ate large meat meals, they wore heavy uniforms, and, a major problem all their time in India, they drank alcohol in even larger quantities than at home, not only from the impressive stores that they brought with them, but also various local brews which were very potent and sometimes poisonous.

Independent travellers and merchants on their own business would adopt Muslim dress as suitable for the climate, and to avoid attack by thieves by not looking like foreigners. But there was always the hazard with loose clothing that

> the habitual fear of entanglement, and facility with which the dress can be laid hold of, tend to take off from a man's boldness.

But many of the Company's merchants, as well as the soldiers, continued to wear their accustomed heavy clothing to maintain the dignity of their rank and position, particularly when on deputation to the local rulers. The refusal to adapt clothing to the climate, in spite of protests from the surgeons, was to be a continuing cause of incapacity, and even death, from heatstroke.

Once the survivors had recovered from the voyage, they began to demand large quantities of meat. This might be difficult in areas under Hindu control where the taking of animal life was forbidden. But in Muslim areas there was no shortage of fresh meat, for the Muslims ate meat, except pork which was forbidden. The English made the most of this, and there was:

> more Flesh killed for the English alone here [Surat] in one Month, than for a year for all the Moors in that populous city.

It took them time to realize that huge meals increased the likelihood of illness in hot weather. Attempts were then made to persuade the men to eat lighter local food in smaller quantities, particularly in the middle of the day. But the strict diet of the Hindus seemed meagre and not at all to their taste:

> as these Indians are extremely fastidious in edibles, there is neither flesh nor fish to be had amongst them ... onely rice, Butter or Milk, and other such inanimate things.

It was better with the curries and pilaus with meat of the Muslims, which were considered to be more health-promoting. But, in general, the local food and spices were only additions to the normal English meal. Indian food was only tolerated by the merchants when there was nothing else to be had. Their men had less choice. Even when there was plenty of fresh meat, they were expected to eat rice like the local people. On one or two days a week they were served *kitcheree* of 'small peas and rice'. This was regarded by the authorities as nourishing, but the hungry men cursed what they called the 'banian days'.

The English were familiar with the stench of the drinking water on board ship, and it was some time before they learned that the water in India could cause disease. They still believed that water from the Thames had special properties of lightness and resistance to corruption (p.39). They found that the Ganges had a similar reputation. Its water was sweeter, and 'one pint weigheth less by one ounce, than any other water'. To the Hindus the Ganges was holy, and all who drank it were cleansed of their sins. To the Muslims it was the most wholesome, so that the Emperor and all who could afford it ensured that they had a constant supply. Trustworthy servants collected the water directly from the river, sealed it in casks, and sent it on camels to the Emperor, wherever he might be. For Hindus the water was collected by brahmins, sealed by the chief priest, and sold to the wealthy who would use it at festivals or for guests at the end of a meal. But among its other properties, the Ganges always contained a large number of partially-burned floating bodies. Wealthy Hindus burned the bodies of their dead and scattered the ashes on the river. If a family was too poor to buy enough wood,

> they only sindge their faces and throw them into the River, of which sort lay a multitude all alonge the water side, putrifieinge and stinckinge, loathsome to behold.

The English thought that the Indians must know how to 'render water wholesome by some concoction'.

The earliest Indian civilizations knew how to make alcohol. At first there were no restrictions, and drunkenness was common. The classical medical texts describe the beneficial effects of alcohol in moderation and the diseases that result from excess. Recipes are given to relieve the after-effects, including small quantities of the same type of wine that caused the drunkenness. By the time the English arrived, alcohol was ritually forbidden to Muslims and they took opium instead, often in large doses. But there was always a great deal of drinking in private by Muslim noblemen. No high-caste Hindu would taste alcohol or sell it, although they gave it to their fighting elephants. But the making and drinking of alcohol was widespread among the lower castes and the hill tribes. The English were accustomed to heavy drinking and they brought a large quantity of liquor with them. The Emperor Akbar gave them a licence to make alcohol, saying that 'to prohibit them the use of it is to deprive them of life'. When supplies ran out they grumbled at the restrictions that limited the amount that they could obtain locally. The penalties for making arrack[11] were very severe – 'death to the partie and destruction to the howse where it shall be found.' It could only be made in secret and it was of poor quality. Any European encampment was soon surrounded by sellers of the local brew, which was usually

> a spirit as harsh and burning as that made from corn in Poland, and the use of it to the least excess occasions nervous and incurable disorders.

The English found that they could gain favour with Muslim noblemen by gifts of European wines and spirits, for 'the Moores prize them farre above theyre owne'. Jahangir (Emperor 1605-27) was addicted to alcohol and opium from the age of eighteen. He established the custom of drinking at his Court, although no-one was allowed to drink without his permission. William Hawkins (p. 29) became one of his favourite drinking companions. Sir Thomas Roe in Agra in 1615 was handed a jewelled cup of 'mingled wyne more strong than ever I tasted, so that it made me sneeze'. The nobles at the Court were sometimes commanded to drink, and it was an offence to refuse. If Jahangir got so drunk that he forgot that he had given permission, those who drank were heavily punished, usually by whipping, which sometimes resulted in death.

Gifts of liquor and heavy drinking were often necessary to ensure trading concessions. The English, although renowned for their hard drinking, were surpassed by the Dutch. But once, when the English invited the Dutch to a feast, 'the Hollanders tooke the licker so well that they were sicke on it most part of the weeke following'. This delayed their sailing, to the great advantage of the English who got ahead of them in the local markets.

It was difficult to get the English to reduce their accustomed intake of alcohol. At first this was a disciplinary matter. Drunkenness at sea was always severely punished. On land, it played a large part in giving the English a bad reputation:

> the disordered carriage of the most parte of our men ... would make a mans eares to tingle to repeate the villanies that was done by them.

One man killed a calf, 'a slaughter more than murther in India'. A diplomatic disaster was narrowly averted, and the man was publicly punished. Others 'made themselves beasts, and so fell to lewde women ... that in shorte time manie fell sicke.'

It was soon recognized that alcohol carried severe health hazards in the heat, increasing the severity of the common local diseases (agues and fluxes), especially in men who lay out on the ground at night in a drunken stupor:

> more English fell in Hindostan by the intemperate and injudicious use of ardent spirits than by the sword.

Some of the English, particularly the more senior, recognized the dangers, and began to see the benefits of drinking water.

But many remained convinced that the regular intake of alcohol was essential for their continuing health, particularly in the tropics. It was also safer than most of the drinking water available. Alcohol had always been highly regarded for its medicinal value. It was prescribed for many diseases, with exact recommendations for the best sort of liquor and its dose. Wine was generally favoured. The Directors were well aware of this and took care to provide adequate supplies for all ships and factories. Even arrack might do good if not taken to excess. Toddy (sap of date- or coco-palm) was a pleasant white wine when drawn, and was only dangerous when it was fermented which was preferred by the men. But it was cheap and good for 'griping of the Gutts'; it promoted the flow of urine, so that it alleviated the (bladder) stone, 'the tyrant of all maladies'. When Peruvian bark (quinine) became available for the treatment of fevers (p. 88) it was found to be so bitter that patients refused to take it unless it was made into a tincture with wine. Alcohol, usually in the form of rum, could be used to preserve fruit juice for the prevention and treatment of scurvy. It was, with opium, the only available analgesic and anaesthetic.

The common local diseases – 'agues' (various forms of malaria) and 'bloody fluxes' (dysentery from polluted water) – were familiar in their European forms, but now of greater virulence, exacerbated by the heat, spreading rapidly through the small isolated close-knit communities of traders and soldiers. The resulting high mortality and the struggle to survive and trade in sometimes hostile conditions meant that the survivors were always under severe stress. The small factory left at Bantam in 1602 on the first Company voyage was in continual trouble from sickness, assaults by the natives and quarrelling with the Dutch. There were only twelve men in the garrison, and these, often ill, had to keep constant guard and to turn out at all times of night for various alarms, particularly fire attacks. Even when allowed to sleep they were disturbed by nightmares, 'we being continually in feare of our lives, some of our men were distract of their witts'.

The Company sent out surgeons with each voyage, but the early factories were often short of surgeons, who died at the same rate as their patients. It took at least a year before a replacement could arrive from England. The surgeons had little or no experience of treating tropical diseases, and they brought contemporary European methods with them – heroic bleeding and purging, and the use of mercury, often in large doses. They tried their standard remedies but their patients often found them not only ineffective or dangerous in the altered conditions but contrary to the practice of the local physicians:

> [the] chirurgion's dyet of Burned Wine to men sick of the flux is by the physitions of this country held rather poysonous than cureable, which some of us in our own experience have found true.

The surgeons might want to continue to prescribe European drugs but these were often in short supply, having been lost or damaged on the voyage. At Fort St. George there was no harbour until the eighteenth century; cargoes were unloaded into small boats which had to cross three lines of surf, and there were many accidents. Even if the drugs arrived unspoilt, they might decay in the heat. Many of them were found to be ineffective:

> drugs far fetcht and longe kept, applied by an unskilfull hand, without consideration of temperature of the body by alteration of climate produce small or contrary effects.

The merchants were quicker than the surgeons to realize that Indian drugs might be more effective for Indian diseases:

> wee doe hold safest for an Englishman to Indianize and, so conforming himself in some manner to the diett of the country, the ordinarie physick of the country will bee the best cure when any sickness shall overtake him.

The English were, at first, impressed by the apparent good health of the Indians and their freedom from some of the diseases familiar in Europe. The use of oil on the skin was seen to have a protective function, allowing the naked Hindu to expose himself to heavy rain without illness. The 'Mussulmans' were 'of good stature, with few hunch-back'd or lame among them'. The Hindus seemed to have more old people than the English, and this was attributed to their temperance in eating and drinking. They were 'all very strait', with none deformed, owing to their habit of lying flat without a pillow, and to not being 'laced or girt'.

They were particularly struck by the women and children. The women delivered their babies so easily that

> while they are labouring or planting they go aside as if to do their Needs, deliver themselves, wash the child, and lay it in a Cot or Hammock, and return to work again.

The children were hardy and strong,

> They bring up their Children naked till seven years of Age, nor do they take much care to teach them to go, but let them tumble about the Ground as much as they will, as soon as they are Born ... and by degrees they come to walk as straight as ours do, without the torture of Swathing-bands or Clouts.

But they recognized that the women and children that they saw were mostly from the poorer classes. When they learned more of the conditions in the houses of the rich they found that women of the higher castes led very restricted lives with no exercise in monotonous surroundings.

The English were also amazed by the bodily cleanliness of the Hindus who washed often and thoroughly so that their feet were as clean as their hands. This, with the use of sweet oils to anoint their bodies, meant that their company was 'very savoury'. The women were always neat and clean, washing at least once a day and again after excretion and 'the companie of their husbands'. Their houses and privies were regularly cleaned by the halalcores (sweepers), 'soe that there is seldome any ill savor in their howses of office'. There were many 'publick Bagnio's and Hot-Houses', which were free.

But in spite of the Indians' general appearance of good health and cleanliness, their lack of vigour and their leisurely life-style were often criticized. It was assumed that the excessive heat was responsible for this. Indians were subject to the plague which 'sweeps away many thousands when it comes into great populous cities', and their commonest diseases were 'the bloody flux and burning feavers'. But they seemed to be free from 'ordinary agues and those two torments, the gout and the stone'. Even though venereal disease was common it was 'not of so virulent a character, or attended with such injurious consequences, as in other parts of the world'. This was thought to be due to the dry air and to the patients going to the baths to sweat out the disease, and to the frequent drinking of tea which produced 'perpetual perspirations'. The Indians' apparent relative freedom from disease made the English think that they had some natural immunity or very effective methods of treatment (p. 74 f.n.5).

But they were struck by the relative unconcern of the Hindus for human life compared with their devotion to animals. This was based on the belief that reincarnation might bring back the human soul in animal form so that harming an animal might endanger a man's relatives. The secretary to the English traders in Surat kept and nourished a large snake which was said to contain the soul of his father. The best human souls would return to be lodged in a cow, the glutton would go to a pig, the lustful to a monkey, the cruel to a tiger, the shrew to a wasp, and a light woman to a fly.

There were no hospitals for humans, but a number for animals of all sorts.[12] The English at first assumed that this custom extended over the whole of India. But all their early expeditions landed in the area of Surat and Cambay, where the Jain religion was predominant, with its ban on the taking of life in any form (p. 43). The Jains wore masks to prevent them inhaling insects, and they had the paths swept clean before them. Travellers arriving at night in a strange village might have difficulty in finding their way about,

> as the Banians burn no candles for fear that Flies and such other Insects might be destroyed thereby ... and they make some difficulty to piss on the Ground, for fear of drowning the Fleas and other Insects which might lye in the way.

The hospitals and their attendants were maintained by public charity. When the animals were cured, they were 'if wild, let go at liberty; if domestick, given to some pious person who keeps them in his House'.

One mile from Surat was a hospital for cows, horses, goats, and dogs. Nearby was a separate hospital 'for the preservation of Buggs, Fleas and other Vermin, which suck the Blood of Men'. A poor man was paid to stay there all night for them to feed on, but he had to be fastened to the bed 'lest the stinging of them might force him to take his flight before the Morning'. Not only wounded and diseased animals were admitted but also those bought 'from Christians and Moors that they may deliver them from the cruelty of

Infidels'. There was a special area for goats bought from Muslims to prevent their ritual sacrifice. Young English merchants found that an easy way to make money was to go out into the fields and pretend to shoot. Devout Hindus would then bribe them to go away.

Although there were no hospitals, there were many practitioners — all physicians. There were no surgeons, but there were barbers who let blood and applied leeches, and whose skills at shaving and 'champinge'[13] were soon recognized. The English, at first, found it hard to distinguish the folk-practitioners from the classically trained — they all used similar methods of treatment. For most diseases the main remedy was fasting. The public bathhouses (hummums) provided welcome relief from the exhaustion of the hot weather and treatment by cupping and sweating for a number of diseases such as 'the barbiers' (beriberi, p. 97).

Since the English surgeons were obviously inexperienced in dealing with the local diseases, the English turned to Indian physicians who would naturally have greater skills and more efficient drugs. The shortage of English surgeons led to the employment of Indian physicians. This became official Company policy in the first half of the seventeenth century, and Indians reached the payroll as 'salary for the Banian Doctor'. Some officials in India even suggested that, if local practitioners were available, English surgeons might not be necessary, for the diseases 'are most familiarly cured by the natives to whome nor means nor skill is wanting'.

As well as recommending fasting, Indian physicians used a wide variety of herbal medicines which they collected from the local countryside. It was generally held in the sixteenth and seventeenth centuries that each country was provided, by a benevolent deity, with the drugs and herbs necessary to treat the diseases of that country:

> God is so merciful that in each land he gives us medicines to cure us. He who causes the illness provides the medicine for it.

It became Company policy that Indian diseases were best treated by Indian methods. The English surgeons set out to learn as much as they could about Indian drugs. They studied the local plants for their medicinal properties, and began to include them in their prescriptions.

The country people seemed to make little use of physicians, 'fearing them more than the disease'. In some areas there were 'hardly any physicians except for the Kings and Princes':

> As for the commonality, when the rains have fallen and it is the season to collect plants, in the mornings you see mothers

of families going out from the towns and villages to collect
the simples which they know to be proper for the diseases
which occur in a family.

In the towns there were men sitting in the market-place or at a corner of the street, handing out potions or plasters.

They first feel the pulse, and when giving the medicine, for
which they take only the value of two farthings, they mumble
some words between their teeth.

The English surgeons would have found much that was familiar. There were many similarities between sixteenth century European medicine and classical Indian Medicine (p. 13). Their first medical contacts were more with folk-medicine than with the classical systems, and they condemned some of the extravagant rituals and dependence on magic, thinking that this was typical of all Indian Medicine. But European medicine still had a great deal of magic in it with a belief in witchcraft and sorcery, and they could accept that supernatural forces might be involved in any successful cure. They noted the medical customs of the areas they visited, and recorded the local remedies for the local diseases, particularly those remedies that they had tried out on themselves and found to be effective.

One of the charges of the Company to their ships' captains and merchants was to search for, and bring back, medicinal products. The voyage in 1614 had instructions, on reaching the Cape, to collect the root *nangin* (ginseng), highly esteemed as a restorative, and therefore very valuable. With the success of the first English expeditions, the import of drugs into England from outside Europe increased from 14 per cent in 1588 to 48 per cent in 1621, and 70 per cent by 1669. The majority of these had come from India and the East Indies:

... a purging medicine newly found out in the East Indies,
and thence brought to us ... Doctor Haruy useth it in Saint
Bartholomews Hospitall.

Once their small factories were established on the coast, the English sought to extend their trade by moving inland. There they came in more direct contact with the ruling classes and with the classical systems of Indian Medicine, and they were able to use their surgical skills to obtain trading concessions. They still had a great deal to learn about the need to modify their European habits, and the simple precautions that would allow more healthy living in the tropics. Gradually they became acclimatized.

Notes

1 Jainism developed in parallel with Buddhism from the fifth century BC.

2 The highest of the four Hindu estates; second is the warrior or ruler; third, the trader; fourth, the outcast, untouchable.

3 'foreigner', first used by Hindus for the Portuguese.

4 Hindu traders, especially in Gujerat. The term was applied by the early traders to Hindus generally.

5 It was not until the nineteenth century that all Company trainee civil servants had to pass a test in an Indian language.

6 Employment in the Company was sometimes a way of getting rid of young rebels, 'the madcaps sent out to die, getting into drunken scrapes'. Robert Clive (p. 101) was packed off to India in the mid-eighteenth century; his family was seriously concerned that he might be mad.

7 This would lead to medical problems when high-caste Hindus were recruited to the Company's armies in the eighteenth century (p. 121).

8 *sati*, 'virtuous woman' (Sanskr.), was not made illegal until 1829 (p. 186).

9 Factor – a general term for a merchant – originally the third class of the Company's (civil) servants: Senior Merchant, Junior Merchant, Factor and Writer.

10 The introductory handshake, instinctive to a westerner, was contamination to a brahmin, and standing to urinate (instead of squatting) was like a dog and therefore unclean.

11 arak, 'perspiration' (Ar.) – a general term for distilled spirits, commonly from the date palm or unrefined sugar.

12 Animal hospitals (referred to as 'Banian hospitals') were still to be found in some of the towns of western India in the late nineteenth century.

13 Massage by kneading and inunction of oils, and twisting the joints until they cracked, but without pain.

Chapter Six
Acclimatization

By 1634 the Company had 140 merchants in 17 factories in India and three in Persia, under the control of the President and Council in Surat. They relied on the local rulers for protection. But the accession of Shah Jehan, a bigoted Muslim, in 1627 brought general disorder. They needed to build their own forts to protect their trading. There had been factories on 'the Coast' (Coromandel, east) since 1611. In 1639 a grant of land was made on the site of the present-day Madras, and Fort St. George was built. In 1641 it had a garrison of thirty-five.

The Fort was close to the Portuguese settlements, and the Directors asked whether this was safe. The reply was that the Portuguese men were no longer a threat, but the women could be a danger,

> so that divers of the English soldiers are married, which must be tolerated, or the Hot shots will take liberty otherwise to coole themselves.

With their forts the English were able to offer protection to their employees. Part of the land to the north of Fort St. George was given over to the 'washers to whiten their callicos being the only part protect with ffort Ordnance'.

But it was Bengal, with the river traffic up and down the Ganges, that had always been the centre of trade for India. The Portuguese had had a settlement there since 1518. It would become the most important part of India for the trading interests of the Company and, later, the centre of government of British India. In 1632 the Portuguese were again defeated at sea, and their influence on the east coast began to decline. After an embassy to Shah Jehan in 1650 the English were given their first licence to trade in Bengal. This concession may have been helped by a Company surgeon, Gabriel Boughton, who was summoned to Agra in 1645 to treat one of the Emperor's daughters. She had been severely burned while trying to save her favourite dancing woman whose clothes had caught fire. The woman died but the princess survived under Boughton's care. He is said to have asked for, and been granted, preferential treatment for the Company in Bengal.[1]

Company surgeons, in the early days, were required to serve in any capacity, and, when necessary, to double as factor, steward, chaplain or even combatant officer. They were always liable to be sent on political missions to local rulers, and they were expected to use their medical knowledge and surgical expertise to gain access to powerful officers at Indian courts. The Indians also used their medical men as diplomats and confidential messengers.

Indian rulers and nobles, as well as recruiting Europeans for their armies, would employ European surgeons, as their own practitioners had little experience. Pitre de Lan, a young Dutch surgeon, had been part of the Embassy from Batavia to the King of Golconda (c. 1654). He was left behind at the request of the King who

> always suffered from a pain in the head, and the physicians had ordered him to be bled under the tongue in four places; but he was unable to find any one willing to undertake it.

De Lan was asked if he could bleed well, and he replied that it was the least difficult part of surgery. He was told that he must not draw more than eight ounces. Basins of gold had been prepared to catch the blood. When the basins were weighed by the King's physicians the blood was found to weigh eight ounces exactly. Hearing of his success, the ladies of the Court asked to be bled also, but 'more from the curiosity they had to see him than for any need they had to be bled'.

Fear of being poisoned led the rulers to take stringent precautions:

> He expects the Physician should lead the way, take Pill for Pill, Dose for Dose, of the same which is administered to him.

They rewarded their doctors well if the treatment was successful, but there were severe penalties for failure. An Italian surgeon, employed by the Dutch (c. 1615), undertook to cure the King of Butan's eldest son of 'distraction of his wits'. He was warned of the dangers but he prescribed opium in wine, and the patient died in the night. The Italian was cut to pieces by the King's sons.

All Europeans were credited with special medical skills, and there were many quacks and adventurers. Nicolao Manucci from Venice, who was in India for more than fifty years from 1656, started as an artilleryman with no medical experience, and turned himself into a prosperous physician by his quick wits and audacity. But when he first set up as a doctor, 'my heart beat fast, for then I had had no experience.' In Delhi, he entered the service of the eldest son of the Emperor Aurangzeb. He had to undergo tests before he was accepted. He was given a pulse to feel in an arm put through a hole in a curtain, with the presumption that this would be one of the royal ladies. He correctly reported that it was a man's arm. Then he was sent a vessel full of urine, with a request to make a diagnosis of a sick princess's illness. He noticed a greenish tinge, and correctly concluded that it was cow's urine. Finally he gained the confidence of the prince, and was given freedom to practice. He became so popular with the princesses and their ladies that they were bled by him regularly once a month. For this the arm was put through the curtain, but covered so as to leave 'one little spot uncovered, about as wide as two fingers'. Like all the other physicians he was conducted through the seraglio by eunuchs, with his head and body covered down to the waist. Later, as a special privilege, he was allowed to enter uncovered. He found that the women often feigned illness simply to have a chance to talk to him.

Every English factory was supposed to have at least one surgeon, but the continuing high mortality often left them with none. Surgeons might be recruited from newly-arrived ships, or, in an emergency, from any European with a little medical training. Every surgeon was entitled to bring an apprentice with him who might be posted as 'the surgion' when there were no qualified men available. On the fourth voyage (1608), three men were accused of murder. Two were hanged. The third, 'the drommer, beeng younge, was repreeved, havinge some skill in surgerye', but he died of dysentery soon afterwards. Some men came out as private soldiers but with a smattering of medical knowledge. They were allowed to purchase their discharge and practise medicine.

Indian practitioners were appointed to fill the vacancies, and this continued throughout the seventeenth century. Official reports refer to 'our Banyan doctor' and 'the Indian doctor'. Outside the main factories there were increasing numbers of junior merchants in isolated posts, as well as individual European merchants and travellers who were wholly dependent on Indians for their medical care and were appreciative of the benefit they received. John Marshall, a factor in 'Pattana' (1668-77), had very little access to any European medical advice. He learned from local practitioners about Hindu medicine with its three humours and the medicines needed to counteract their imbalance. He described the Hindu expertise with metals and minerals and their use in medicinal preparations. He and his colleagues often tried, and proved the efficacy of, Indian remedies. The Hindu doctors had prescriptions, often of multiple ingredients, for dropsy, gout, stone and the French pox. There were also purges and remedies for snake- and scorpion-bites, fevers, wounds and bruises, toothache, disorders of the guts, worms, barbeers (beriberi), ague and epilepsy. The cautery was often used:

> A man in India must be very regular in Eating, or he will fall into some incurable Distemper; or at least such as must be cured after the Country fashion with fire; Experience having shown that European Medicines are no use there.

The Portuguese had been the first to compare the pattern of diseases of Indians and of Europeans in the East, and of their response to treatment:

> The Physitians that go out of Portugal into those parts, must at first keep company with the Indian surgeons to be fit to Practice, otherwise if they go about to cure those Distempers, so far different from ours, after the European manner, they may chance to Kill more than they Cure.

The English surgeons soon had their first experience of treating Indians. They were in increasing demand from the poor who would attach themselves to any European in the hope of some medical relief.

> Any man who could call himself a physician bore a title to which in this country the best passport is of very inferior consideration.

A convoy of the Company's goods from inland to Surat in 1614 was joined by many poor travellers.

> Our chirurgeon (whome we intreted for in case of such accidentes) ... was forced to spend all his store broughte with him upon the poore people, which came to shelter themselves under our protection, whereby manie of their lives and goodes were saved.

They found that their Indian patients were easier to treat than their own countrymen, 'debauched in Brandy and Aqua vitae':

> Illnesses in the Mogul country are very easy to cure, owing to the heat, which causes perspiration and thus relieves the patient.

Indians did not stand the harsh European treatments so well, but they were accustomed to the heat and had 'no Aqua vitae of their own, but only such as we use now and then to treat them withal'.

The English were impressed by how well the lightly-clad abstemious Hindu tolerated the fierce climate. They thought that this must be due to the vegetarian diet:

> for many of the Gentus,[2] especially the brahmans and the banyans ... eat nothing whatever that has been alive, not even eggs, or red vegetables, which they shrink from as blood.

The surgeons learned that this abstinence, from meat in particular, was regarded as a positive factor in avoiding and treating illness. The principle was familiar to them from their practice of Galenic medicine (p. 13), with its emphasis on control of disease by diet. They began to recommend abstinence as a way of keeping healthy in the heat and as a method of treatment, particularly for fevers.

> Their practice differs essentially from ours ... a patient with a fever requires no great nourishment; the sovereign remedy for sickness is abstinence; nothing is worse for a sick body than meat broth, for it soon corrupts in the stomach of one afflicted with fever; a patient should be bled, only on extraordinary occasions, a brain fever, or inflammation of the chest, liver or kidneys ... these modes of treatment are successful in Hindustan, and the Mogol and Mahometan physicians ... adopt them no less than do those of the Gentiles, especially in regard to abstinence from meat broth.

Abstinence was then applied to other conditions such as severe injuries, bloody fluxe, and *mort-de-chien* (cholera).

The surgeons had learned on the voyage the dangers of blood-letting in scurvy. They began to recognize that Europeans after any length of time in India were likely to be so weakened that they could not withstand the loss of blood, and that mercury should only be used with great care. As they started to treat Indians they found that the same precautions were necessary. But they noticed that Indians seemed to be less susceptible to the diseases that affected the English, and they concluded that this was partly due to their abstemious habits. The lightly-clad Hindu, who could carry heavy loads in the heat, who lived on vegetables, and, in the higher castes, was forbidden alcohol, was compared with the thick clothing and uniforms of the English, their meat diet and their heavy drinking.

The frugal habits of the Hindus were commended by the surgeons, reinforced by the chaplains:

> a wise man will here accustom himself to the pure and fine water, or to the excellent lemonade, which costs little and may be drunk without injury ... the happy ignorance which

prevails of many distempers is fairly ascribable to the general habits of sobriety among the people.

But these exhortations lost some of their effect when it was found that Indians, although their wounds healed quickly, withstood injury and loss of blood less well than Europeans.

Over-eating and drinking was the rule among the English. A common table was always part of the strong corporate life of the relatively small numbers of English in each settlement. In Surat in 1628 there was a substantial Company house with a community of twenty-six including the surgeon. They were starting to introduce Indian food, but this was often in addition to their accustomed diet:

> Our Dyett heere for the most part is such as wee have in England, fine bread of Wheate, Beefe, Mutton, Henns, pigeons, dressed after our owne manner by English Cookes. Sometymes wee have this countrey wilde fowle, Antelops, and perchance wildeboare; but ordinarilie wee have dopeage [a Persian savoury dish – probably curry] and Rice, Kercheere [grain boiled with rice and salt] and achare or pickled Manges.

There was also less alcohol:

> Our stronge Drinck is Racke [arrack], like strong water, next a kinde of beere made of Course Sugar and other ingredients, pleasant to the taste and wholesome, but many tymes water.

The soldiers, under orders, persisted with their heavy uniforms with thick tunics and constricting leather equipment. Some of the younger factors and writers, particularly the 'griffins' (the new arrivals), behaved in a foolhardy way in the heat, regarding it as a sign of weakness to make concessions. Noblemen travelling independently might feel that their status required that they should swelter in their finest clothes, although warned that this might make them more liable to attack. The chaplains at first kept to their long black cassocks, and 'stewed in our own moisture', so that sudden changes of temperature were likely to cause serious illness. They found that a compromise was necessary: 'we all kept to our English habits, made as light and cool as possibly we could have them.' The senior merchants were quicker to 'indianize' their dress. This was not only for comfort but also for protection, so as to appear as little conspicuous as possible, particularly when travelling.

> Wee live after this Countrie manner in matter of meate, drincke and apparrell ... going out, a *shash* [turban] on our heads, a *doopata* or white lynnen scarfe over our shoulders (this in Summer and Pummering [wool] in Winter); then a fine white lynnen Coate, a girdle to binde about us, breeches and shooes, our swords and daggers by our sides.

In the Company House in Agra in 1632 the rooms were carpeted with cushions to lean on in public as well as in private, 'after the Customs of this place, sitting on the ground att our meat or discourse'.

Gradually they came to realize that there was less need for food in the heat and that heavy meals led to illness. They could even get used to rice in place of bread:

> according as one is habituated to the Air of the Country, one accustoms one's self also to the use of Rice, and grows out of conceit with Bread. Rice is wholsome, creates little Blood and little Excrement, and does not cause Vapours.

It also had medicinal properties – 'in agues and other distempers, it tempers and purifies the blood.' But many of the men continued to demand the heavy meat meals they were accustomed to. Meat was plentiful, and sold in every part of the cities, but it was not to be trusted unless it was 'dressed at home'. Mutton and beef were 'heating, flatulent and difficult of digestion'. Buffaloes were cheap, but 'often cause dysentery', and

> the Wild Oxen ingenders Imposthumations in the same parts, and as painful as those that are contracted from lewd Women.

Attempts were made to get the men to eat more Indian food, and in smaller quantities, especially in the middle of the day.

They began to pay more attention to the quality of their drinking water. Ganges water still retained the local reputation that 'it never becomes bad, and engenders no vermin', but this was outweighed by the number of dead bodies floating in it. They learned that the Dutch never drank water unless it had been boiled, and 'as for the native inhabitants, they have been accustomed to it from their youth'. They found that Ganges water caused diarrhoea, and all who were forced to drink it boiled it. But they were impressed by the Indian methods of cooling water and other drinks. For the Emperor, ice was brought from the Himalayas. In ordinary houses ice made in the 'Indian way'[3] was used in drinks all the year round and was sold all over the cities. The English found it dangerous to drink large quantities of very cold liquids when overheated. In the summer,

> when the wind was like standing in front of a hot furnace, many die merely from the heat, because they are tempted to drink milk or cold water. For this reason they nearly all drink hot water.

The dangers of drinking water only enhanced the natural inclination of the English for alcohol. Their surgeons, although sometimes as drunken as their patients (this improved from the early eighteenth century), began to see the connection between over-indulgence in liquor and the incidence of tropical diseases – not only in causing disease, but also in making it more lethal. The dangers of the local toddy and arrack were repeatedly stressed in official warnings – 'prejudicial to the health of the men, making them intoxicated and debilitated and very much impair their Memores'. The common danger was lying out in the open at night in a drunken stupor. Fevers and fluxes soon followed, and the mortality was high. The recommendation was 'to keep warm under a cover and sleep out the fermentation'. Seamen and soldiers could be troublesome when drunk, and they were best left alone to 'vent that Fury, by breathing [lancing] a Vein or two with their own Swords, sometimes slashing themselves most Barbarously'. Some of the English copied the local habit of taking the 'herb Dutra' [*datura*, stramonium] with which the Muslims laced their drinks. The English found that it helped 'in their pleasant Frolicks', but if taken to excess it could lead to them becoming *amouki* or 'running a Muck'.

Abuse of alcohol continued to pose major problems throughout the English (later, British) period in India. Nearly every health report from the earliest times referred to the relation of alcohol to disease. Frequent edicts were sent out by the Court of Directors with little effect. The Company in India made repeated attempts to control drunkenness by regulating the supply of alcohol and the places where it could be obtained. Orders were issued that no locally-made arrack was to be sold to any servant of the Company, all punch-houses[4] had to be licensed by the Governor, and each man was rationed to half-a-pint of spirits. No liquor was to be drawn after the eight o'clock curfew when everybody was to go home. Anyone caught illegally making or selling liquor was fined, and the liquor confiscated for medical use in the hospitals.

An important reason for founding the early hospitals (p. 69) was to provide a place for the soldiers to be confined, so that the surgeon could ensure that they were prevented from obtaining liquor, legal or illegal. The surgeons' health warnings were reinforced by the chaplains who repeatedly urged the men to copy the piety and abstemiousness of the Hindus,

> [who] hating gluttony, and esteeming drunkenness, as indeed it is, another madness; and therefore have but one word in their language, though it be very copious, and, that word is *mest*, for a drunkard, and a mad-man.

If there was any drunkenness among Indians, it was 'only among the dregs of the people, and then not very often'. But alcohol was regularly drunk by Muslim noblemen. The Emperor Jahangir, a heavy drinker, was succeeded by his grandson, Shah Jehan (Emperor 1627-57), who was not a drinker himself, but gave full liberty to his nobles. This was reversed by the ascetic Aurangzeb (1657-1707), who also compelled all Christians, except physicians and surgeons, to leave the city, and to move one league away. There they were permitted to prepare and drink liquor, but not to sell it. Anyone selling liquor in the city was hunted down and condemned to lose one hand and one foot. These laws were gradually relaxed, while the nobles continued to distil liquor privately in their own houses as they always had done:

> ... as a Remedy against Sorrow ... they generally drink the Strongest, and to make it more Heady they put in Nux vomica, Hempseed and Lime. Wine is too cool for 'em, they must have some Brandy, and the stronger it is, the better they like it.

As well as presents of strong liquor, the English would entertain Muslim officials who envied the Christians their sumptuous feasts and could sometimes be persuaded to overlook the prohibition on pork. The Company Agent invited the local Governor to drink wine with him. When this was well received it was arranged that, at the next visit, food should be served. This included pigling, which was referred to as 'kid'. It was greatly appreciated, and 'much good feeling was engendered to the favour of the Company'.

In spite of the recognized health hazards alcohol retained its important place in the treatment of disease. It was regularly prescribed, usually in the form of wine, particularly for fevers (p. 87). Sallow-water (brandy extracted from a type of willow) was used in Persia for all fevers, and many Europeans endorsed its efficacy. Alcohol was also regarded as essential to counteract the depression induced by the harsh and often isolated conditions, the threat of disease, and the death of companions. When the Governor of Surat tried to ingratiate himself with the Directors by his economy, the factors complained bitterly that he was depriving them of

> the comfort of Europe Liquors, which the Company's Bounty yearly bestowed, for the people's principal delight is to see new drinks arrive ... they contribute to health; and the majority fear that they will not survive for the remainder of the year if they do not receive these supplies.

In an attempt to reduce the high levels of disease, the English, for a short time, followed a policy of 'indianization', based on the Indians' apparent immunity to some of the local diseases. It was thought that if the blood of a European could be made more like that of an Indian he would be more resistant to Indian diseases. This had been started by the Portuguese who ascribed their high mortality to the local diet which was new to them. Those who escaped an early death then lived in reasonable health. Thus they concluded that their blood had been changed.

> Upon this erroneous principle, they adopted a most fatal method of seasoning people to these unhealthy climates. By repeated bleedings they took away as much blood as they supposed to be contained in the body.

They then fed them exclusively on Indian food. But the Portuguese were notorious for their vigorous blood-letting.

> The Physicians are great bleeders, insomuch that they exceed often Galen's advice, *ad deliquium* [to fainting], in Fevers, hardly leaving enough to feed the Curents for Circulation; of which Cruelty some complain invidiously after Recovery.

The English copied this idea but felt that it was only necessary to starve the men without bleeding before filling them with local food, and that this combined with local remedies would give them the same resistance as the Indians. There were soon objections even to this practice when it was seen that the English were more resistant to injury and loss of blood than Indians. This was attributed to the meat in their diet. It was also seen that the Indians' 'resistance' was highly selective, applying mainly to fevers,[5] and to a lesser extent to fluxes. Their generally poor living conditions with under-nourishment and over-crowding made them more susceptible to epidemics such as cholera and plague.

In the plague epidemics in Surat in the last quarter of the seventeenth century the Indians were much more severely affected than the English. In a bad season there were 300 deaths a day, although the city seemed to go on unchanged. The Indians said that God was with the English because none of them were affected even though their servants died. The English thought that this was due to the 'generous wines and costly Dishes ... the strength of that Aliment whereon we feed', although in spite of this many of them were languid, feeble, and less vigorous than the Indians. Nevertheless they were spared, and the chaplains concluded that

> there may be reason for the Pious opinion of the Indians that the Almighty displays an extraordinary Power in our Preservation.

The small English garrisons, depleted by sickness and the reputed attractions of service under the Muslims, made repeated requests to the Directors for more men and medical supplies:

> We have had a very unhealthful and sickly tyme amongst us ever since Christmas last; hardly a man that hath not been visited more or lesse, some of us 4 or 5 tymes over. We could intreate you to supply us with tenn Englishmen to serve here as soldyers, for Mortality and Moores Campp hath taken all away to 25 persons, whereof 4 or 5 are continually sick with the miseerie of the time.

The sickness rate was always highest at the changes of season and in the newly-arrived recruits. There were many complaints that the men who had to carry out heavy duties in severe conditions had not enough wages to obtain warm billets or to buy the supplies they needed when they were ill.

At first there was no separate accommodation for the sick, who had to remain in their billets around the town where it was difficult to supervise or treat them. In the factory they were a dangerous source of infection. It was soon recognized that they had to be isolated from the main living area. This would reduce the risks of infection, and allow supervision. It was always expected that the normal Englishman, unless carefully supervised, would eat and drink more than was good for him. In extremes of temperature this could be fatal. In a hospital with sentries on the gates, the sick could be isolated and their intake of food and drink strictly controlled by the surgeons.

The merchants pleaded with the Directors to provide funds to build hospitals. They used the argument that it would save money by reducing the need to send out so many new recruits to replace the ones who had died. They were sure that this would please their masters. When permission was finally given it was accompanied by detailed instructions to ensure the utmost economy at all stages. The first hospitals were opened at Fort St. George (1654), Bombay (1676), and Calcutta (1707). These were for Europeans only. At first only unmarried men were to be admitted; married men were to be looked after at home by their wives. The patients had to pay their own expenses, and if they could not do this they were not to be admitted. The local community was expected to pay for the upkeep and daily running of the hospital. There were constant grumbles from the civilians at the great expense of all this when most of the patients were Company soldiers. Finally the Directors were persuaded to take over the funding, and it was agreed that all needy patients should be admitted free whether they were soldiers or civilians.

Many of the new arrivals were already unhealthy when they reached India bringing infections with them and making them vulnerable to the local diseases. They were often of poor quality to start with,

> from the gaols and Hospitals whereby one third dye in the voyage and infect the ship; half of which do arrive, are put into the Hospital and many never come out.

But if they survived the first onslaught of tropical conditions and diseases it was seen that there was a fair chance that they would become 'salted', allowing them to stay on in relative safety. The older and more senior of the Company's servants, making concessions to the heat and becoming more temperate in their eating and drinking, found that the climate seemed to be 'suited to men from forty up to old age; but it is very unhealthy for young men'.

The authorities came to recognize the advantages of a period of isolation for all new arrivals in India. At first they were concerned to protect them from the hazards of the local liquor by keeping them in hospital and putting guards on the gates. Later, regular systems were introduced for quarantine of any ship suspected of carrying infection, and for acclimatization of all newly-arrived troops, although a military emergency might mean that they would have to be sent straight up-country.

The English were beginning to see the risks of some of their habits. There were simple measures that they could adopt to conform to the climate, as recorded by M. Bernier:[6]

> There was a great mortality among the Dutch and English when they first settled in Bengale; and I saw in Balasa two very fine English vessels, which had remained in that port a twelvemonth in consequence of the war with Holland,

and at the expiration of the period, were unable to put to sea, because the greater part of the crew had died. Both the English and the Dutch now live with more caution and the mortality is diminished. The masters of vessels take care that their crews drink less punch; nor do they permit them so frequently to visit the Indian women, or the dealers in *arac* and tobacco. Good Vin de Grave or Canary and Chiras wines, taken in moderation, are found excellent preservatives against the effects of bad air, therefore I maintain that those who live carefully need not be sick, nor will the mortality be greater among them than with the rest of the world.

But the mortality was still high. More of them died in September and October than in all the rest of the year, and this continued throughout the seventeenth century. By the end of September 1690 the chaplain in Bombay had buried twenty out of twenty-four passengers and more than fifteen of the crew of the ship that brought him to India. The English were now familiar with this seasonal pattern of disease and the dangerous times at changes in the weather when they would be exposed to extremes of temperature which would bring on fevers and fluxes. They were unprepared for the famine of 1630-2 that nearly destroyed their settlements in western India.

There was little margin for survival among the poor, and a year of drought and poor harvests was usually followed by famine, and then often by an epidemic. A widespread epidemic with a high mortality would mean that there were not enough people to till the fields, leading to a poor harvest and further famine. The English were involved in the famines of the seventeenth century with no responsibility for their relief. They were affected as severely as the Indians by the lack of food and by the high mortality in the subsequent epidemics.

Drought in western India in 1629 led to the great famine of 1630-2, one of the most severe in the seventeenth century. One of the English survivors, Peter Mundy, on his first tour of service with the Company (1628-34), gave a full account:

> the Famine it selfe swept away more than a Million of the Common or poorer Sort. After which, the mortalities succeedinge did as much more amongst the rich and poore.

On his journey from Surat to Agra in 1630,

> all the high waies were so full of dead bodyes, that wee could hardly pass from them without treadinge on or goeinge over some.

He passed through towns that were almost deserted,

> where wee were much troubled to find a roome convenient for our little Tent, by reason of the number of dead bodyes that lay scattered in and about the Towne.

His small caravan was everywhere increased by people attaching themselves to him in the hope of escaping to a better area and seeking security for the journey. They would scrape in the dung of the travellers' animals in the hopes of finding some undigested grains. Around Agra, people were selling their children, or giving them away, to richer Indians or Europeans,

> to any that would take them, with manye thancks, that soe they might preserve them alive, although they were sure never to see them againe.

When the rains came they were so unusually heavy that they destroyed any remaining crops. Business was at a standstill with the dispersal of the surviving traders and Indian weavers. There was no transport for any goods that could be bought, and all journeys became increasingly hazardous with large marauding bands lying in wait.

Three years later, in March 1633, on his way back to Surat, Mundy described the depopulation that was apparent everywhere. In Surat the small colony of Company servants had been almost wiped out:

> there were but few liveing of those I left heere att my departure, the rest dead with the Mortall Sicknesses that imedeatly followed the famine.

Fourteen of the twenty-one alive in 1630 were dead, and three more were dying, 'there being Scarce one Man in all Suratt-house able to write'.

The English surgeons had many opportunities to observe the clinical effects of starvation:

> I have examined some dying of Famine, who told mee that within their bodies they were hot, but without cold, especially on their Belly and privy parts. They are very thirsty

and hungry, and are so feeble that can neither go nor stand, nor scarce stir any joynt. They have no pain in their head, but a great one in their Navill. Their urin is very red and thick like blood, and excrement like water, which runs often from them, but but little at a time.

They recognized that it was dangerous to over-feed starving men, and that they should at first be given only small quantities of rice.

The English saw no efforts being made at any time by the Mogul authorities, either to alleviate the effects of the famine or to dispose of the bodies. Mundy noted that the King, with his army, was in the neighbourhood, and all available supplies were commandeered for him. As Mundy's party travelled through the region they noticed that the areas of famine were separated from unaffected areas by only relatively short distances, but that there was no transport to carry food to the starving, even if the officials had been willing to make the arrangements – all the transport was being used for the army. There were no arrangements for the disposal of the dead – rotting corpses lay everywhere. If there were too many on the river bank, rich men hired sweepers to pull them out to the middle of the river and launch them downstream.

The official Indian accounts claim that the Emperor not only remitted taxes in the affected areas but gave money to the poor and hungry, and directed his officials to set up centres for the free provision of food. But there was no official distribution of food to the poor. The authorities had handled the crisis by ordering their agents to buy up all the available grain. Even in areas where there was more food,

> people new dead and others breathing their last with the food almost att their mouthes, yett died for want of it, they not haveinge wherewith to buy, nor the others so much pittie to spare them any without money (there being no course taken in this Country to remedie this great evill, the Rich and stronge engrossinge and takeinge perforce all to themselves).

The Company's preoccupation with trade meant that the effects of famine were measured by a tally of the number of weavers in the area. In a later famine, 'an Account of the Number of Looms in the Company's Bounds' showed that there were only 531, compared with 1000 the year before,

> which is a Plaine Demonstration how severe the famine has been that 469 has Died and sold themselves and gone to other Places in so short a time.

Notes

1 In 1715 William Hamilton had similar success in gaining favours for the Company by his treatment of the Emperor Farrukh (p.101).

2 Gentoo/gentile – originally used by the Portuguese for Hindus, as opposed to 'Moors' (Muslims).

3 Porous jars covered with wet cloths and exposed to a draught in the early morning.

4 The popular drink was punch, which was cheap; *panch*, 'five' (Hindi) – made of the five ingredients; sugar, lime-juice, spice, water and arrack.

5 The relative resistance of Indians to 'fevers' (malaria) and their poor resistance to physical injury may have been partly accounted for by sickle-cell anaemia and thalassaemia. Patients affected by these diseases, now common in India, which are known to have existed from very early times, suffer from malaria less frequently and less severely than the unaffected, and their children survive malaria better.

6 François Bernier, a French physician, was in India from 1656-68 in the service of a son of the Emperor Shah Jehan for whom he translated into Persian the works of Harvey and Descartes.

III
THE RISING POWER OF THE COMPANY 1680-1780

Chapter Seven
Increasing medical experience

As the Company recovered after the famine, and trade improved, the English steadily extended their activities in India. The Portuguese no longer posed a threat, and the Dutch influence was largely confined to the East Indies. The English were now less dependent on the goodwill of local rulers for trading concessions. As the advances in medicine in Europe were transmitted to India by better-trained physicians they were increasingly critical of Indian Medicine and what they came to regard as its out-dated and 'unscientific' practice.

The Company was becoming more prosperous, and making increasing contributions to the wealth of the nation at home. In 1640 they were required to sell their stocks of pepper to the Crown on credit. Charles I at once resold it for £50,000. After the large profits of the early voyages there were some bad years in which no dividend was paid, but by the end of the seventeenth century the average annual dividend was 25 per cent. Trading was interrupted again by the confusion of the Civil War at home. Cromwell's support was obtained in 1657, and trade began to improve. But the Emperor Shah Jehan died that year, and the civil war that followed in India temporarily stopped all trading. The Company got a new Charter from Charles II, and he gave Bombay to the Company in 1668.[1] The city rapidly increased in size and authority and soon took over from Surat as the headquarters of trade in western India. James II renewed the Company's Charter in 1686, promoting Bombay and Madras to Regencies under the King.

The Emperor Aurangzeb (1657-1707) had rebelled against his father and came to the throne after defeating and killing his two elder brothers. Unlike his predecessors he was violently anti-Hindu. Towards the end of the seventeenth century his power began to wane, leading to the gradual disintegration of the Mogul Empire in the eighteenth century. European observers noted that the Empire was becoming vulnerable to attack by any competent army. The loss of central control by the Empire put the English under heavy pressure from aggressive local rulers. Attacks by the Mahrattas were repulsed by small Company forces. The Directors were always urging avoidance of military action and trying to economize. But their servants in India were determined to fight to defend what they believed to be their just trading rights — the transition from 'flattery and propitiation to forts and righteous aggression'.

They continued to build up their forts. By 1670 Fort St. George had a garrison of 300 English; Bombay was being fortified at the same time. From 1677 the Bengal factory under Job Charnock was being continually harassed by the local ruler. Charnock was at first defeated and the English had to leave Bengal. Aurangzeb offered peace as he wanted the English to keep the pilgrim route secure across the Arabian Sea. In 1690 Charnock returned to found the city of Calcutta. Fort William, which was established there in 1700, eventually became the British centre in India. By 1702 the Company had 13 factories (including three in Persia) under the control of Bombay, 14 (including one in China)[2] under Fort St. George, and nine under Fort William.

In England the first of the many complaints about the evils of the India trade were heard. English workers were being put out of work by the import of cheap Indian goods. There were also accusations of mistreatment of Indians. Complaints in England about the political, military and social activities of the Company were to continue intermittently until the final days of the Company in the nineteenth century.

Service with the Company was now more attractive, and the social standing of applicants was rising. Although salaries were still low, the Company's servants received rich gifts every year from Hindu traders, and they were allowed private trading if it did not interfere with the passage of goods back to England. Living standards in India were high. In Surat in 1689 the Company was keeping its servants 'not only in Decency, but Splendor', and the Company House had the best 'accommodations' in the city. At Fort St. George, Company officials were also living in style surrounded by Indian servants and travelling with 'flags, troops and processions'.

Company discipline was strict. Copies of the main rules – the Company's Commandments – were printed and sent out to India. Absence from prayers on the Sabbath or Wednesday mornings, unless on duty, was punished. Swearing and blaspheming were forbidden. Abuse of Indians and drunkenness were punished by putting the culprit in irons. For the soldiers it was laid down that every Sabbath and day when exercising they should 'weare English Apparrell as becoming their Profession'.

Women were now allowed out to India. At first they were wives accompanying their husbands or going out to join their husbands, although some of the husbands were dead by the time their wives arrived. But since European women were scarce in India the widows had little difficulty in marrying again, often to men in senior positions. The Company allowed marriage to English women in India, and gave berths to women 'to go out to gain husbands, which they do (and good ones) and deserve them after the perils of the voyage'. Such good fortune soon became known in England and was the start of the trickle of young women making their way to India in search of rich husbands, which was to become the flood of the 'Fishing Fleet' of the nineteenth century (p.209).

But it was a different matter for the common soldiers and the junior writers and officials. There were no English women to spare for them. There were official edicts and dire warnings from the preachers about contacts with local women, but most of the men had an Indian or Portuguese partner. The authorities were afraid that the men would marry Portuguese women and so be at risk of conversion to Catholicism. To prevent this the Company started sending out women for the soldiers to marry. They had great difficulty in selecting these women who had to pay their own passage. They were not given any allowance, so that on arrival some were found to be destitute, and had to be supported by local funds as long as they remained unmarried. The conditions for these women were in general so unsatisfactory, and the conduct of some of them so outrageous, that many of them had to be sent home.

With more women reaching India increasing numbers of English children were born. In contrast to the good health of Indian children (p. 54) they were a sickly lot with a high mortality in infancy. This was attributed to the women

> living at large not debarring themselves wine and strong drink which, immoderately used, influences the blood and spoils the milk in these hot countries ... the natives abhor all heady liquors for which reason they approve better nurses ... as the Dutch well observe those thrive better that come of an European Father and Indian Mother.

Only about one child in twenty survived, and the survivors had to be sent home. It was realized that there was no chance of building up the English population, and that replacements from home would always be needed.

As the English began to feel more secure and less dependent on Indians, they became increasingly critical of Indian knowledge. They questioned the philosophers and 'classical' physicians about their beliefs and practice, and they were scornful of their lack of learning. Even the brahmins were 'silly, sottish and ignorant'. Benares (Varanasi) might be 'the Athens of India' but the scholars were very indolent. The English were also contemptuous of the people's credulity:

> upon the Hills by Casmere there are men that live some hundreds of years ... every year some of them come down unto the people at Ganges, and do many great Cures; for

whom they have such a veneration that they frequently drink the Water they wash their sweaty Feet in.

The earlier sympathy of the English surgeons for Indian Medicine was changing as new ideas came in from Europe:

On physic they have a great number of small books, which are rather collections of recipes than regular treatises. The [Hindu] physicians follow the ancient books which say a great deal, but tell very little.

The hakims were also criticized. Their methods were to feel the pulse, let blood, and prescribe 'more Hog-wash at one stroke than three mens bellys are able to contain'. The chaplains had extolled the virtues of the abstemious Hindus but now it was seen that their life-expectancy was less than that of Europeans in Europe. The influence of a meat diet remained controversial. Abstinence from meat did not seem to make any difference to the length of life – Muslims lived as long as Hindus – but it seemed to prevent Hindus becoming strong and vigorous. Although their tolerance of extreme heat was enviable they were very sensitive to the cold.

When the weather is cold, the people will not fish at all if they can avoid it; for they have a much greater dread of cold than Europeans have of heat.

The surgeons were now more experienced in tropical diseases, and their knowledge of local drugs and herbs was increasing so that they used them in their prescriptions when appropriate, without having to rely on Indian practitioners. As early as 1621 the Directors were urging that India had drugs 'in far greater quantity, plenty and perfection than here', and that they should be bought locally. The early budgets always included an allowance for 'country' medicines. In 1698 in Madras the bill was £50 per year for European medicines, and the same for 'drugs and medicines procurable in these parts'. Surgeons began to collect specimens from the surrounding countryside either for immediate use or for propagation in physic gardens attached to the new hospitals. Some of the specimens were sent home as whole plants or seeds for further study and possible use in England (p. 239).

Indian physicians, by long observation of local diseases, might be expected to have better success than foreign physicians. This was shown in their management of fevers by cooling (p. 87). But for the flux they did not give anodyne enemas but only astringents, so that the patients suffered torments by day and night. To alleviate the pain they gave opium in doses that would be harmful to a European. Their purges were relatively mild and they did not know of the chemical preparations routinely used by the English so that they were surprised to see

> us Foreigners produce such Evacuations as we do, by the help of such small quantities of Physick.

The English had always put their faith in blood-letting, particularly for fevers. But Hindu physicians were more conservative, aiming to cool the blood with herbs and congee[3] and general abstinence. Muslim practitioners were more radical than the English, bleeding their patients

> not in the trifling manner of the modern practitioners, but copiously, like the ancients, taking eighteen or twenty ounces of blood, sometimes even to fainting.

While Indian practitioners relied on the classical texts, the concept of disease was changing in Europe. The 'humoral' theory was fading as advances in physics and chemistry showed that vital phenomena had mechanical explanations, e.g. Harvey's (1628) demonstration of the circulation of the blood. Sydenham[4] introduced his classification of diseases, and showed that the specific treatment for a disease would remove it from the body rather than restore the balance of the humours. New powerful drugs were being introduced, e.g. cinchona bark (quinine) for the rapid cure of fevers (p. 246). This was also a time of specialized anatomical research in Europe. English surgeons were scornful of the traditional Hindu concepts of anatomy:

> ... yet notwithstanding their profound ignorance, they affirm that the number of veins in the human body is five thousand, neither more nor less; just as if they had carefully reckoned them.

Towards the end of the seventeenth century the Company began to recruit physicians who were better educated than the apprenticed surgeons. They brought with them to India the latest medical doctrines from Europe. These were based on scientific principles which they regarded as far superior to traditional Indian Medicine. This was the start of the general denigration of Indian ideas that would characterize medical thinking in India in the eighteenth century.

The most distinguished Company physician at this time was John Fryer,[5] who was in India from 1672-81. He was appointed 'Chirurgeon for Bombay at 50s. per month' in 1672 and remained in India, with some time in Persia, until 1681. He kept notes of everything that he saw, and his account (1698) included information on religions, customs and folk-lore. He made many botanical observations including medicinal plants. He described scurvy on the outward voyage and once the sick were on shore their rapid recovery by eating oranges and limes.

He was often called to treat patients outside the Company's service – Indian rulers and their families and wealthy Portuguese. Like all medical men in India he was required to combine medical with political skills on diplomatic missions. Requests from Indians for medical help were encouraged in the interests of good trading. He was always told in advance which Indians were to be his patients, but in accordance with local custom he had to postpone the consultation until a 'Lucky Day' as determined by the astrologer. He was once commanded by the English President in Bombay to make an arduous journey into the Deccan to see one of the Mogul's generals, and to treat one of his wives. After elaborate precautions, he gained admission to the harem where the patient was on a bed hung with silk curtains. He was only allowed to feel the lady's pulse by putting his hand under the curtains. The first hand that was presented seemed to him to be perfectly normal, and he said so. Since this was the hand of a healthy slave-girl put to test him, he was regarded with great favour. When the next hand was presented to him 'which demonstrated a weak languid Constitution' he had no hesitation in making a diagnosis and prescribing treatment. The next day he was called again to bleed one of the Governor's wives, 'he being tolerated Four, though he keeps more than Three hundred Concubines'. This time an arm was held out through a hole in the curtain. After she had been bled, the lady showed her appreciation by 'pouring upon her extravasated Blood a Golden shower of Pagods[6] which I made my Man fish for'. According to his instructions, after the successful treatment of the general and his family, he proposed 'an intercourse of Commerce between this place and Bombain'.

Fryer gave a detailed account of Indian Medicine which he had learned from local practitioners. Although he found some things to commend in their system he was critical of what he regarded as their 'Ignorance and malpractice', noting that 'here they will submit to Spells and Charms, and the Advice of Old Women'. He criticized the alchemists 'who cast a scandal on the Noble Profession of Chymistry, to which is owing the true Knowledge of Physick'. He held to the seventeenth century doctrine that each country possessed the remedies for its own diseases. At Surat he learned from an Indian doctor how to identify the various local medicinal plants and their uses. This brahmin doctor came to the factory every day to feel the men's pulses and prescribe the necessary treatment. He had a powder, 'a preparation of natural cinnabar' (mercuric sulphide), which was as effective for agues as Peruvian Bark (quinine).

But Fryer was critical of the Indians' lack of formal training, so that 'Physick here is now as in former days, open to all Pretenders'. He saw a barber treating 'a Bloody Flux' by laying the patient on his back and thrusting with all his strength on the belly before fastening a pot full of earth to it and 'making it fast with a Ligature'. The patient died.

> Even those that are most skilled, have it by Tradition, or former Experience descending in their Families. They are unskill'd in Anatomy ... Chirurgery is in as bad a plight ... Pharmacy is in no better condition; Apothecaries here being no more than Perfumers. In Fevers, their Method is to prescribe Coolers, till they have extinguished the Vital Heat; and if the Patients are so robust to conquer the Remedies used to quench the Flame of the Acute Disease, yet are they left labouring under Chronical ones, as Dropsy, Jaundice, and Ill Habits, a long while before they recover their Pristine Heat.

But he noted the ease with which Indian peasant women gave birth, and he compared this with the problems of English women in India (p. 79).

His contact with Indian Medicine had been mainly through Hindu practitioners, but in February 1676/7 he sailed from Surat to spend several months in Persia where the medicine was entirely Muslim (Unani). Here again, he found that there was no formal licence to practise. There was little knowledge of chemistry or anatomy and no attempt to improve on the classical (Arabic) texts. The seasonal pattern of disease was well recognized. The sudden changes of temperature were regarded as the main cause of disease in men and animals. Their medicines were primitive, and seemed to be prescribed indiscriminately, with one ointment serving for all ulcers whatever the cause. Similarly for

> the Distempers themselves ... asking some frivolous Questions, viewing the Veins of the Hands and Feet, inspecting the tongue, they write at adventure ...

The surgeons' skills were very poor, '... yet they are bold enough with the Blood, where they command Phlebotomy, bleeding like Farriers'. Many of the physicians prescribed unusual diets with the meat of goats, horses, asses and camels, and there were separate shambles for these.

> The fashionable Malady of the Country is a Clap,
> scarce One in Ten being free from it ... so that they
> are not come to Maturity, before they are rotten ...

Almost as common were 'piles' from 'constant being on Horseback' and 'their aptness to Venery, and proneness to make use of Boys'.

> They applaud all Provocatives in Physick, and will purchase them at any Rates; which are sometimes so strong, that they create a continued Priapism ... To divert their Care and Labours, they are great Devourers of Opium ... which they quaff when they have a mind to be merry ... they begin gradually, and then arrive to great Quantities ... by means whereof, without any other Sustenances, they are qualified to undergo great Travels and Hardships: But having once begun, they must continue it, or else they dye.

Back in India, Fryer noted that 'the Diseases reign according to the Seasons', and he recorded the pattern: with the north winds of the dry 'winter' season all bodily functions were improved and there was generally good health; in the 'variable months' were coughs, catarrhs, rheumatism and intermittent fevers, with smallpox in children; in the extreme heat, *cholera morbus* for which 'they apply Cauteries most unmercifully'; in the rains, fluxes, 'Apoplexies, and all Distempers of the Brain, as well as Stomach.' September and October were the most dangerous months. More Europeans died then than in all the rest of the year. Of 80 English men in Surat in 1691 there were only 27 in 1696:

> which common Fatality has created a Proverb among the English there, that Two Mussouns [monsoons] are the Age of a Man.

Bombay was particularly unhealthy. There was no hospital until 1678, 'only a burying-place'. Fryer noted the large staff and elaborate ceremony of the President and other officials, and commented, 'but for all the Gallantry, I reckon they walk but in Charnel-houses.' He condemned the filth in the streets of Surat — 'this City is very nasty by their want of Privies, and their making every Door a Dunghill.' He thought that the quality of the water was important in preventing disease. In Bombay there were no fresh streams, and the water in the city was 'rain, preserved in tanks, which decaying, strain into wells; it was always brackish'.[7]

Fryer had noted the insanitary conditions in Bombay but, of the three larger trading centres chosen by the English in the seventeenth century, only Madras was reasonably healthy. Bombay was known as 'the burying ground of the English'. Calcutta was worse. Bombay and Calcutta had extensive marshes on their landward sides. These were favoured by the soldiers as providing an open field of fire, but they were also ideal breeding-grounds for malarial mosquitoes. In Bombay reclamation of the land was not started until 1721. The unhealthiness of the air was attributed to the local habit of stacking fish round the roots of the coconut trees to manure them. This shut out the sea-breezes and created a most unsavoury smell.

> In the Mornings there is generally seen a thick Fog among those Trees, that affects both the Brains and Lungs of Europeans, and breeds Consumptions, Fevers and Fluxes.
>
> The Water is as bad as the Soil, and the Air nothing better; all which conspiring together, carries off abundance of Sailors and Soldiers.

Against this continuing mortality – high even by contemporary European levels – the first hospitals (p. 70) were judged to be a success. The Directors congratulated the staff at Fort St. George for 'preserving the Healths of our Men'. In 1677 Bombay reported that only 15 soldiers had died, compared with 100 the year before, and they attributed this to the new hospital. It was also noted that the lowered death-rate meant that fewer replacements would be needed which would save the Company several hundred pounds a year. But death was often due less to the climate than to the irregular habits of the men and lack of attention when they were sick.

> For to persons in a flux ... which is ye country disease, strong drink and flesh is mortall, which to make an English souldier leave of is almost as difficult as to make him divest his nature.

Once they were in hospital nothing could be brought in without permission from the surgeon. Indian doctors were still employed as physicians. In 1689 the President in Surat provided 'an Indian Doctor of Physick, and an English surgeon'. Any drugs required were charged to the Company 'so that the Factors have all that is necessary'.

No hospitals were provided at this time by the Indians for their own people, and there was no official treatment of Indians by the English apart from specific employment by Indian rulers. Missionaries gave what help they could to the poor. The first Indian troops were recruited by the Company in 1677 but no special arrangements were made for their medical care which was left to their own practitioners.

The English surgeons had always used Indians as dressers, and unofficially had trained them in various medical tasks. In the new hospitals most of the nursing and the chores were done by Indians. In emergencies a few soldiers would be detailed off to look after their comrades. Training of Indians now became more formal, particularly in the compounding of medicines. There were many testimonials by the surgeons to the skill and care of their Indian dressers. In 1690 listed on the payroll at Fort St. George were two 'physicians', father and son, who had served the Company for over fifty years. The son had acted as assistant to his father until he became competent, when he was listed as 'physician'; both were entrusted with making up prescriptions. These early training schemes gradually became regularized, leading to the full medical training of Indians in western medicine in the middle of the nineteenth century (p. 199).

But Bombay, in spite of the success of its hospital, remained very unhealthy with:

> Fluxes, Dropsy, Scurvy, Barbiers [beriberi] which is an enervating of the whole body, being neither able to use Hands or Feet, Gout, Stone, Malignant and Putrid Fevers which are Endemial diseases.

Calcutta, on the worst site, did not have a hospital until 1707. It was a fine building but it soon got the reputation of a place to be avoided:

> ... a pretty good hospital at Calcutta, where many go in to undergo the penance of Physic, but few come out to give an account of its operation.

In England the outbreaks of plague in the seventeenth century led to the use of 'searchers' to see every case of death and to send in the results, particularly from plague, to the Parish Clerks. From these, 'Bills of Mortality' were issued. The first rudimentary public health measures in India included, in 1677, instructions from the Directors that similar records were to be kept and sent back annually to London.

The commonest cause of death was **fever**, thought to be due to bad air – 'malaria'. Mosquito-borne malaria was common in England in the seventeenth century, and the surgeons were familiar with 'ague'. But the varied and severe forms that they encountered in India were regarded as separate diseases to which they gave separate names, such as 'Bengal fever', 'Jungle fever', 'malignant' or *pucker*[8] fever (very violent), 'bilious fever' (with copious vomiting) and 'salting fever' (affecting the new arrivals). These were all different forms of malaria, and they all carried a high mortality.

It was generally agreed that fevers arose from marshy ground, and that the decay of animal and vegetable remains gave rise to a gas which was unidentifiable and only known by its effects on man. This gas was produced in small pools and tanks (reservoirs) and was rendered harmless by direct sunlight. It could also be arrested by gauze. It was trapped by woods and jungle, and was particularly concentrated in the dew at night. It was set free when the land was cultivated, and there was a high incidence of fever at the end of the rainy season when the farmers were starting to prepare the land. The poison was usually inhaled, but it could occasionally be taken in through the skin, either from the atmosphere or by bathing. There was debate as to how far it could be carried by the wind and what physical features, such as woods and lakes, could protect from it. Ships that anchored well away from land remained free of fever.

Many of these observations on the production and spread of this 'bad air' were correct and can be correlated with the natural history of the mosquito (p. 114), but the link was not made until the end of the nineteenth century (p. 220). Mosquitoes were regarded as just one more of the pests of India. There were many complaints of the nuisance they caused: 'the greatest Pest is the Mosquito, who not only wheals, but domineers by its continual Hums.' Elaborate precautions were taken for protection:

> fine Calicut-Lawn thrown over their beds ... long Breeches to their toes, and Mufflers on their Hands and Face, and a servant to keep them from them with a fan, without which there is no sleeping.

Indian physicians treated fevers by strictly limiting the diet, with only water to drink and congee for sustenenance. This regime was at first commended by the English – it was like the one recommended by 'the ancient Physicians' (Galen). The European prescription of 'Jelly-broath' seven or eight times a day with new-laid eggs might actually contain more nourishment than the patient was accustomed to. Congee was easily taken by the patient who often found strong broth repugnant. The patient was moved to as cool a place as possible, his head was shaved, wet cloths were applied to his head and body, and copious cold drinks were given. But wine was indispensable for Europeans. Care was needed not to cause too much excitement but if it seemed to be doing good the dose could be increased to two bottles of claret or port in twenty-four hours.

This regime was overtaken by the introduction of quinine in the form of Cinchona bark, which reached Europe from Peru in the middle of the seventeenth century and proved specific for 'malarial' fevers (p. 246). The patient was first cleansed with emetics and purges, and mercury was given in the form of calomel (mercurous chloride) every 4-5 hours. The value of bleeding was debatable. European practice was to bleed vigorously in the early stages of a fever. In India this had to be modified in patients already broken down by the climate. The powdered bark was then given, either continuously or timed to prevent relapses, depending on the views of the surgeon. The bark was extremely bitter and it was usually given as a tincture in wine. Opium was given with it for general relief. Even so it could be nauseating, and some patients refused to continue after the first dose; they always did badly. There were also a number of traditional Indian preparations which were in vogue from time to time.[9] These might have to be used when bark was scarce, and some of them were reputed to be at least as powerful as the bark, which often deteriorated on the voyage.

After fevers, **fluxes** (dysentery) were the commonest cause of death. Even in seasons when other diseases were less virulent, there were always cases of diarrhoea with a steady mortality. These varied in severity from 'flux' (diarrhoea) to 'bloody flux' (tropical dysentery) to 'cholera' which was often rapidly fatal. These terms were often used indiscriminately. If the disease was 'true' *cholera morbus* it must have been invariably fatal. There were many instances when a violent diarrhoeal illness was described as 'cholera' but the patient recovered; these were probably examples of tropical dysentery.

Cholera was endemic in India but did not appear in Europe until the early nineteenth century. The upper Ganges basin, the worst area affected, had always been the site of religious festivals, usually in March and April, and these were often followed by epidemics among the pilgrims who spread it widely as they returned home. The epidemic in Goa in the sixteenth century was described by da Orta (p. 24). A change of diet was liable to provoke the distemper:

> changing all our victuals and drink upon a sudden, it changeth our flesh into another nature; and if a man be not very moderate and careful, it is a thousand to one if he catch not some disease or another presently, the bloody flukes being the rifest, which is seldom helped and killeth a lusty strong man in ten days.

But the main cause was thought to be bad water. It was worse in the winter when the water had become less wholesome from the amount of flood-water.

An important contributory factor was the men 'going open, and cold in the stomacke' when overheated.

In the treatment of diarrhoea there was little distinction between relatively mild cases and those severe enough to be labelled 'cholera'. Europeans were always more difficult to cure than Indians because of their 'debaucheries in Wine and Aqua vitae'.

> The common people of the Indies have no other remedy against this distemper, but Rice boyled in water till it be dry, they eat it with Milk turned sower, and use no other food as long as the distemper lasts; the same they use for a Bloody Flux.

The English added opium — 'the Pills of Laudanum, without which the Patients will have but little rest'. When treating Indians, many of whom were addicted to opium, they found that they would tolerate doses that would be dangerous to Europeans. It was important to avoid changes of temperature, particularly the night dews. The patient wore a flannel shirt with a flannel bandage round his belly. A long shawl was recommended for the officers but if they could not afford this, flannel was just as good. All surgeons agreed on the value of mercury (calomel) every 3-6 hours in all varieties of dysentery. 'As soon as there is free ptyalism [salivation] the patient is safe for that time', and 'every judicious practitioner employs it.' It could prevent and treat the infection of the liver that occurred in some cases (amoebic dysentery) (p.90). Their faith in the efficacy of mercury in diseases of the gut and liver in India led to the belief that there must be some 'indigenous and local poison, or miasma, peculiar to the country'. Mercury was regarded as specific for this as for syphilis. But they recognized that Indian diseases were different from European, and that care was needed in transferring this treatment to other countries (p. 248).

In some of the cases of 'cholera' there were clear descriptions of overwhelming attacks with rapid prostration and death in a very short time. This was *cholera morbus* or 'mort-de-chien' (p. 27 f.n.8). Here 'the early restoration of balance in the circulation' was essential by warm baths, cordials such as warm punch, with opium, calomel, and frictions with hot flannels.[10] The Indian treatment that attracted the most interest was burning the soles of the feet:

> They heat a Peg of Iron about half as big as ones Finger red hot, clap it to the sole of the Patients heel, and hold it there till he be no longer able to endure it; so that the Iron leaves a mark behind it.

This was sometimes accompanied by:

> binding the Patients head so fast with a Swathing-band, as if they had a mind to squeeze out his Brains; they do the same with his Back, Reins, thighs and Legs, and when the Patient finds no good of this Ligature, they think him past cure.

If there was much colic, the iron might also be applied to the site:

> so that those who have the good fortune to recover carry the signs of the Fire afterwards on their Belly.

English surgeons might have thought this treatment ridiculous before going to India, but, in the confusion over the definition of 'cholera', they saw enough successes to convince them of its efficacy. As they moved inland from the coastal areas, however, they found that 'the miraculous effects of this treatment were little known'.

If they made no clear distinction between cholera and the other causes of severe diarrhoea, they also did not differentiate the two types of dysentery — bacterial (tropical dysentery) and amoebic.[11] It had long been recognized that the liver could be affected in cases of dysentery, and that sometimes in the terminal stages it was destroyed by abscesses. The general term **hepatitis** was used to cover this and other disorders of the liver. In Europe hepatitis could be an acute illness but this was rare in India. Chronic hepatitis, the 'Endemic of India', developed more slowly and, if not treated, abscesses would form in the liver. This was amoebic dysentery, with subsequent infection of the liver, and it was much commoner in the tropics than in temperate climates. Once the liver was affected, the mortality was 50 per cent. The abscesses were at first sterile, but if they were opened surgically or burst spontaneously secondary infection was almost always fatal. Treatment was with laxatives, inunctions of mercury twice a day over the liver, calomel or mercurial pills, blisters and opiates. If this failed the only remedy was to return to Europe. Once in Europe some recovered, but others lingered on in chronic ill health. In 1660 ipecacuanha was introduced into India and was found to be effective in some of these cases.[12]

Plague, spreading from China, had reached England in 1348. There were recurrent epidemics, but with lessening intensity, until the last in 1655. The overall mortality was 50 per cent. It was recognized as highly contagious and particularly dangerous to surgeons who were advised to wear gloves of oiled silk when attending the sick. Physicians survived by carefully avoiding all contact with patients.

The first account of plague in India was in 1616 when the symptoms were accurately described by the Emperor Jahangir. In the next eight years it spread everywhere in northern and western India. It was always noticed that plague followed the finding of dead rats. The Vedas had warned people to desert their houses 'when rats fall from the roofs above, jump about and die'. The Indian custom of treating the walls and floors of their houses with cow-dung was thought to protect against plague. The disease carried a very high mortality. Of a small group of English, seven died in nine days, including the surgeon. They had a high fever and 'broad spots of a black and blue colour on their breasts'; they all died within twenty-four hours of the onset. In 1616 in Agra there were one thousand deaths daily in the worst three months. The Muslim rulers, believing that all illness came directly from God, rarely took any measures of prevention or control. Similarly, since the sick were not to blame, they were not segregated.

Experience in India led to modifications in treatment. All agreed that bleeding, strong purging and emetics were ineffective. Sweating and blisters to the buboes[13] (to extract the poison) had been recommended by the College of Physicians. However, sweating was found to kill the patients from exhaustion, and some who sweated least survived. The protective function of the lymphatic system was now better understood, and there was no harm in leaving the buboes to resolve. Mercury was useless – it was possible to catch plague while under salivation for venereal disease. Frictions with oil, another old remedy, were not only useless but dangerous to those applying them.

Smallpox was common all over India. It was believed that the disease was controlled by the goddess Sitala Mata. She is displayed riding on a donkey with a basket of grain on her head, a pitcher of water in one hand and a broom in the other. When she shakes her head the grain spills and each one turns into a pustule. If she uses the water to clean the spilt grain the patient will survive; if she uses only the dry broom, he will die. Treatment often consisted only of sacrifices and prayers to the goddess. Smallpox was well-known to the English but they expected that the disease would be less serious than in Europe because the climate would keep the pores open and help to expel the poison. In the coastal areas they found that the patients were left out under the trees with a little congee beside them but no further care until they recovered, but they mostly died.

As the English had, as yet, no responsibility for treating Indians they were not as concerned with the disease as they would be later (p. 173). But they learned of the Indian practice of inoculation.[14] This was carried out more in Bengal than in other parts, and they were told that it had been practised there 'since time out of mind'. One account stated that it had been known for 150 years, started by a physician 'which secret he had immediately of God in a dream'. The inoculators used matter from the pock of a person who has the disease in a favourable way ... they then dip the point of a needle in this matter, and with it prick ... several times in a circle, on the fleshy part of the arm ... the fever comes on about the fifth or seventh day... generally lasts three days, and then goes quite off.

The English noted that nearly every Indian who caught the disease 'in the natural way' died, but that the inoculated usually recovered.

Venereal diseases were already well-known in Europe. Syphilis had reached its maximum virulence in the early sixteenth century and maintained this throughout the century. It was prevalent in the East before the English arrived. Da Orta, in 1563, had reported that 'all these islands and China and Japan have this *morbo napolitano*.' It is possible that the 'large pox' was known in the East from at least the tenth century when the Arabs were using mercury for its treatment. In India the Portuguese were regarded as the source, and syphilis was referred to as 'Phiranga Rogi' (foreigner's disease) by Indian physicians. It was one of the commonest diseases in the Portuguese hospital in Goa (p. 25).

Every port carried the risk of venereal disease, and many travellers were infected before they reached India. In Madagascar (a regular call for watering and re-victualling) the disease in the natives was as common as in Europeans. Their only treatment was a 'broad red hot Iron' applied to the soles of their feet, producing an ulcer which they kept open for 30-40 days 'to evacuate the malignant Humour'. In Persia there was 'scarce One in Ten being free from it'. In India it was common in the coastal towns, and greatly increased by the number of foreigners, particularly the Europeans. Inland there was less disease and this was attributed to the temperance and cleanliness of both sexes — they 'wash the parts of sex three times a day'. Prostitution carried no stigma; the profession was hereditary. Prostitutes were legally entitled to privileges such as exemption from certain taxes.

Later, to protect English troops, a committee at each main centre once a month inspected 'such dulcineas as may be resident within the bounds of the cantonments'. The diseased were sent to small hospitals which offered them treatment without coercion. Soldiers with venereal disease were charged extra for their treatment in an attempt to discourage their activities (p. 118). The English blamed 'the climate, which derives to the bodies living in it no great disposition to Chastity'. Recurrent attacks were common, and repeated courses of treatment were needed. The men made no attempt to conceal the disease and some had had it three or four times. Since it was not lethal when treated in time it was feared much less than other diseases. It was agreed that syphilis was much less dangerous in India than in Europe. The continual perspiration meant that, if the disease was treated early, it could be completely cured. When a ship left port, especially if prize-money had been shared out, there were always a number of venereal patients. They could all be treated without complications and some of them even gained weight. One officer, reporting sick to escape duty, was given calomel pills. He fed the pills to the doctor's hens; all their feathers fell out but they then became the finest birds in the neighbourhood.

The standard treatment was with mercury and bleeding, purging and sweating. The efficacy of mercury had long been known, given either internally as a pill or externally by pulverizing it between the hands and rubbing it into the skin (p.247). It was brought into general use as the disease reached its height in the sixteenth century, and its abuse was soon widespread: 'every horse-leech and bawd now upon each trifle will procure a Mercuriall flux.'[15] John Woodall was well aware of the dangers of overdosing with mercury, and he warned all his apprentices that the margin between curing and killing was small (p. 21).

Recognition of the toxic effects led to trials of many other drugs. Opium in large doses, guiacum, and China Root (*Smilax glabra*) and sarsaparilla (*Smilax officinalis*) brought in by Chinese traders, were widely used in India. Another local remedy was ripe mango: 'they make them break out, and cleanse the blood, and salivate to the height of mercurial.' There were other attempted cures. The English noted that Persians did not eat much poultry:

> ... suspicious of the Ill Practice of their own Nation, who fancy Diseases gotten of Prostitutes are drawn out by buggering of them ...

In China, for the same reason, no European would eat a duck unless it had been reared by him.

The English found that the Indian remedies were less effective than mercury, and they preferred to put up with the unpleasant side-effects in the hope of a more certain cure. Even if the disease was not completely cured it could be kept under control with mercury and they learned to live with it.

Some of the diseases they encountered were less familiar. Around Cochin on the west coast they saw people with one or both legs hugely swollen, and sometimes other parts such as the scrotum. They named this condition **Cochin Leg**.[16] When they found the deformity in people living near the Mount of St. Thomas on the east coast, the Christian traders thought that it must be a judgement on the descendants of the murderers of St. Thomas.[17] The locals thought it was due to 'drinking bad water, to which, as we to the Air, they attribute all diseases'. The swelling caused surprisingly little trouble. Some of them had 'legs as big as most Mens middles', and to the touch 'they felt just like a Spunge'. But they could run as fast as horses. Dutch men and women were also affected, and the men with a silk-stocking, shoe and buckle looked ludicrous – they would have been better in Asiatic dress. There was no treatment. In the nineteenth century there were some successful operations to remove an enormously enlarged scrotum (p. 196).

The **Guinea-Worm**[18] had been described by the Portuguese from their experience in Brazil. The English came across it as soon as they reached the Persian Gulf where they found 'a Plague of Wormes' among the inhabitants. The worm, found most commonly in the legs, could be as long as 'the treble string of a violin'. The victims knew all about the disease which they thought was caught from the drinking water. They treated themselves, winding the worms out of their legs round a twig. They knew that this had to be done slowly and carefully to avoid breaking the worm and causing complications. In India, also, the drinking water was recognized as the problem. The worm had to be kept moist with rose-water, and nourished with milk and butter or a 'poultice of the Patient's own Ordure' to keep it alive. If it died or broke in the process of winding it out there was great pain and swelling. The English debated whether the disease was due to a living animal since, after extraction, it might not move. One surgeon offered a reward to any hakim who would extract a worm whole. At an operation in the surgeon's house an eleven inch worm was extracted from a patient's back. There was no doubt of its vitality:

> a young gentleman of the Civil Service was so disgusted at the horrible appearance of the reptile twisting and writhing during the extraction, that he was obliged to leave.

Indians had always believed that the disease was due to a living animal. If it was superficial they cut down on it and extracted it. If it was more deep-seated they would wait for it to appear, and then draw it out slowly day by day. Europeans often called in Indian doctors, and the treatment was usually completed without complications.

The earliest travellers and traders had reported the expertise of the Indians in the treatment of **snake-bite**. The English, at first, copied the Indians in their dread of snakes in general, believing that:

> some of the snakes of the Indies are so dangerous, especially the green ones, that death is instantaneous; but in the rest there is time to administer antidotes.

This was reinforced by wandering mountebanks. The performer would let himself be bitten by his 'poisonous' snake, the part would swell convincingly, and he would be cured by secret oils and powders which were then sold to the crowd. As the English gradually learned more about the natural history of the snakes of India they began to differentiate between the relatively few that were poisonous and the much greater number that were harmless; some snake-bites were rapidly fatal but most cases recovered however they were treated. They became increasingly sceptical of the harmful effects that were reported after many snake-bites, having come to recognize 'the notoriously deep dread of the natives of the bite of every reptile', and that many of the symptoms were due to a 'passion of fear'. In some holy sites the local people were not afraid of cobras, claiming that they were friendly unless provoked. But most Indians were terrifed of snakes.

At first every surgeon and quack had his certain remedy. All the early accounts of snake-bite reported successful cures with Indian remedies. Da Orta's favourite for all poisons was bezoar (p. 242). Best of all for snake-bite was the 'famed Stone of Cobra' (Pedra de Cobre) (p. 243); this was sure to draw out the poison. Snakes were so common in India that many Europeans

> carry always about them one of these Stones inclosd in a Heart of Gold, fixt to a Golden Chain which hangs about their Necks.

If there was no stone available the wound was scarified and cupped to draw as much blood as possible. A root, Pao de Cobra, was frequently used. It had been discovered in Ceylon by watching the mongoose which anointed itself with this root before a fight with a snake or if it had been bitten would seek out this root in the forest, eat it, and recover completely. Ammonia (a few drops in a wine glass of water every 2-3 hours) was a popular remedy; although it was not specific, it helped in cases where the poison was potentiated by fear. For scorpion bites the Indians used a burning coal held over the wound to draw out the poison. They also recommended an oil made from scorpions. If this was not available, the scorpion that bit you should be pounded up.

By the end of the seventeenth century most of these remedies had been tried by the increasingly experienced English surgeons and found to be ineffective. The first systematic accounts of the snakes of India by Company surgeons were published towards the end of the eighteenth century (p. 220).

Indians were famed for their skill with **poisons** long before the first traders arrived. There was the legend of the Prince of Cambay who, as a boy, had been fed poison regularly by his father to make him immune:

> when he wishes to destroy any great personage he makes him come before him stripped and naked, and then eats certain

> fruits ... and spurts it out upon that person ... so that in the space of half an hour he falls to the ground dead ... every night that he sleeps with a woman she is found dead in the morning.

When the English reached the East Indies they found that the natives were adept at poisoning. They were told that the King had little poisoned arrows which he blew through a pipe to execute his enemies, and that death occurred very rapidly by this method so that even if surgeons were standing by the poison was too quick for them.[19] They found enough evidence that poisoning was common to make them very wary. Some of them came to believe that they were being slowly poisoned over a long period of time. They were careful not to offend the locals, particularly when eating or drinking with them. When drinking punch:

> the rude unpolish'd northern sailor who upsets the wench who makes up the mixture would be well advised to look out for himself.

Since poisoning was so common, Indian rulers took elaborate precautions. There were many suggested remedies and specialists to administer them. Suspected poisons and their possible remedies were tried out on condemned prisoners. Any method that would allow early detection was important. There was a special type of china which cracked when poison was put on it, and it was important to have dishes made of this material. All parts of the rhinoceros, particularly the horn (often believed to come from the unicorn), were highly esteemed and used against all poisons and many other diseases. The English President at Surat was so convinced of this that he exchanged a large silver bowl for a cup made out of the horn, in the expectation that it would 'sweat' if any poison was brought near. Antidotes were highly prized, the most expensive being bezoar stone (p. 242). The small English garrison under siege in their factory at Bantam in 1603 relied on this to protect them. The best Indian antidote was 'Maldivy Coco-Nut'.[20]

The fear of Indians' skill with poisons gradually abated. The English came to think that there was probably no more poisoning in India, and the Indians no more skilled at it, than in any other part of the world, but

> when a Simple Surgeon can give no reason for the State of his patient, and has try'd his two or three Nostrums to no purpose, his last refuge, to save his Credit, is to persuade his Patient some body or other has given him a Dose.

Tetanus (lock-jaw) was a widespread and unsolved problem. The association with wounds and operations was clear, and it was recognized that the affection lay within the spinal canal but the mechanism was unknown. Wounds were opened and filled with spirits of turpentine, but no local application had any effect. Similarly with every sort of medication, including very large doses of opium hourly, although 'the faculty at Madras place great confidence in the liberal use of hot Madeira'. On the hypothesis that irritation from the site of injury spread to the brain by the nerves, amputation or division of nerves was sometimes carried out. Once the jaw was locked treatment was ineffective and all the patients died.

Rabies following a bite from one of the many *pariah* (stray) dogs and jackals afflicted with 'canine madness' was nearly always fatal. Early bold bleeding (until almost pulseless) and mercury were tried. The wound was completely excised followed by cautery or caustics but all measures were useless in severe cases. The Indians also had no remedies and they did not even excise the wound. As with snake-bite, when an Indian had been bitten it was often not certain whether the symptoms were due to the bite or to extreme nervous reaction. The diagnosis was made by offering water which would be refused, and by holding up a mirror at which the patient would shudder and turn away. Effective treatment (with a vaccine) was not developed until the late nineteenth century (p. 220).

Tuberculosis was not common in India, but when it occurred it progressed rapidly and was always fatal. The climate, instead of being beneficial, made the disease worse.[21] Treatment included a blister to the sternum which was then converted into an issue by keeping part of it open with blistering ointment. All medicines were useless – mercury was particularly dangerous. The only hope lay in a sea voyage and a change of climate.

Beriberi, known as 'the barbiers' in India[22], was one of the mysterious diseases in all the early European accounts. It affected mostly the lower class of Europeans after they had been lying drunk in the open air. There was sudden swelling and paralysis of all or parts of the limbs, and sometimes death in a few days. Indians agreed that it was mainly a disease of Europeans, and put it down to 'venereal excess'. The English believed that it was due to the intolerable heat of the land wind blowing on the sleeper. They also thought that it could come from 'being over-physicked for venereal complaints'. It was often confused with scurvy, but it was not thought to be due to any deficiency in the diet as it was no commoner in sudden famines.[23] The Indian treatment was to rub the patient all over with cow-dung and herbs, and bury him up to the chin in hot sand in the middle of the day for as long as he could stand it. Europeans preferred the hummums (public hot baths), sitting wrapped in blankets between two open fires while red-hot bullets were thrown into a cauldron to produce dense clouds of herbal steam. The best cure was to return to Europe or some other bracing climate.

Faced with these lethal diseases, the importance of **psychological factors**, ('the depressing passions') on the incidence of physical illness in the tropics was well-recognized. Those of timid disposition succumbed soonest – the 'pressed men' were particularly vulnerable. The surgeons had always stressed the importance of maintaining a cheeerful attitude at sea as a way of reducing the incidence of diseases such as scurvy. A ship with prize-money would have no troubles and the men would remain healthy. But if things started to go wrong the sickness-rate rose. In India the prevalence of dangerous diseases could induce such a fear of illness that the fear might predispose to the disease:

> if a man arrives in the tropics with the fear that he will die if he gets a fever, he will die. Old hands and good officers can dispel this, and show the value of a temperate life.

The very small number of English compared with the overwhelming masses of Indians gave them a continuing feeling of insecurity. The slow passage to England, taking a year to get an answer to a letter, increased the sense of isolation. Misleading images of India at home might lead to extravagant hopes of making a quick fortune, which were in many cases disappointed. Religion and mental and physical activity were the best shields against all this – 'philosophy and reason are vain, and only efficacious in Europe.' The frequency of disorders of the liver led to the belief that there was a 'sympathetic relation' between it and the mental state, each acting on the other. 'Torpor of the liver', as a result of the heat and the climate, caused mental symptoms which themselves reacted back on the liver. Depression, gloomy thoughts, health worries – 'all can be reversed by rousing the liver'. This usually meant prescribing mercury until the patient was salivating.

The medical information that was now being sent back from India not only added new drugs to the pharmacopoeia but gave good advice to future travellers. This was part of the greatly increased knowledge of the countries in the East that was being collected throughout the seventeenth century, covering political, religious, social and commercial aspects, with details of prevalent diseases and their treatment. By the end of the century some of these accounts had been published, and the authors were able to advise their successors not only how to trade profitably but also how to adapt to the climate to give them a better chance of survival.

Notes

1 Bombay had been acquired by the Portuguese in 1528 and came to Charles as part of the dowry of the Infanta Catherine.

2 Regular trade with Canton established the shipment of tea from China, This would develop into the main trading activity of the Company.

3 *kanji*, 'boilings' (Tamil) – rice boiled for an hour until 'well broken', squeezed through linen, and the fluid given with a little salt.

4 Thomas Sydenham (1624-89), one of the most influential physicians of the seventeenth century, has been called 'the English Hippocrates'.

5 John Fryer (1650-1733), MD Cambridge and, in 1697, the first Company physician to become a Fellow of the Royal Society.

6 One pagoda = approx. 5/- (25p).

7 No major efforts were made to clean up the water supply in India until the middle of the nineteenth century (p. 217).

8 *pakka*, ripe, substantial (Hindi).

9 e.g. a decoction of 'Malabar china' from the bitter leaves of the Veppa tree (*Swietenia febrifuga*), and the kernel of *Caesalpina bonducella*.

10 It was not realized until the nineteenth century that 'restoration of balance' is only possible by intravenous infusion of fluid (p. 221).

11 Amoebic dysentery – infection of the colon by a type of amoeba that is an internal parasite in humans; the infection can spread to the liver. The differentiation of the two types of dysentery was not made until 1828 by Dr (later Sir) James Annesley, a Company medical officer.

12 Ipecacuanha was brought to Europe from Brazil in 1658. It is a powerful emetic, and this was thought to be its mode of action. In 1913 Sir Leonard Rogers IMS showed that the active alkaloid, emetine, has a direct effect on the parasite.

13 swollen lymphatic glands, particularly in the groin and axilla.

14 Inoculation (with the live virus) only started in England in the 1720s. In India, as elsewhere, although protecting the individual, it carried the risk of spreading the natural disease and starting an epidemic.

15 The sign of an effective dose for syphilis was an inflamed mouth and intense salivation.

16 Elephantiasis. It was often confused with leprosy (p.150). Now known as filariasis, caused by thread-like worms whose larvae are transmitted from human to human by mosquitoes. The adult worms live in, and obstruct, lymphatic vessels, leading to enormous swelling of the legs and genitalia.

17 St. Thomas is believed to have been in India from c. AD 52; he was killed near Madras in AD 68 for preaching Christianity.

18 Dracunculus, a long thin worm living under the skin of humans and some domestic animals. The larvae are deposited in water, from which they are picked up by drinking. The worm produces a toxin causing local inflammation and, occasionally, general urticaria. In 1832/3 the worm accounted for 3 per cent of the morbidity of the Bombay Army.

19 It is not clear how many were killed by the poison alone. The power of suggestion must have been very strong, cf. snake-bite (p. 95).

20 Coco-de-mer or double coconut, the fruit of *Lodoicea Sechellarum*.

21 In the twentieth century tuberculosis was widespread, with a mortality second only to malaria.

22 *biribi*, 'jerky gait' (Malay) and *bharbari*, 'swelling' (Hindustani). Deficiency of vitamins of the B group, occurring when the diet consists mainly of polished rice. The heart is affected as well as the peripheral nerves, and sudden death can occur.

23 It was not realized that it takes three months for a deficient diet to have its effect.

Chapter Eight
War with the French

The break-up of the Mogul Empire was accelerated by the civil war that followed the death of Aurangzeb in 1707 (from Delhi Boil, p. 220). Under a succession of short-lived or weak rulers the provinces of the Empire became autonomous. There were repeated invasions by the Afghans, ending in the sack of Delhi in 1757. The collapse of the Empire increased the opportunities for any nation with military power. While the Directors at home continued to urge economy and peaceful settlements the Company in India was using its enlarging army to acquire more land and trading rights and to take over political control from incompetent and warring local rulers.

In 1714 Indian officials in Bengal revoked some of the Company's trading privileges, and an Embassy went to Delhi to put their grievances before the Emperor Farrukh. The merchants with an interpreter and a surgeon, William Hamilton, reached Delhi in July 1715 and stayed for two years. The Emperor was suffering from some disability that was preventing his marriage. Hamilton offered his services, and his treatment was successful in a few weeks.[1] He was rewarded with replicas of his instruments in gold. There is no record that he asked for favours for the Company, but all their privileges were restored.

By the middle of the eighteenth century the Company owned Fort William and six factories in Bengal, Fort St. George and six factories on the east coast and three inland, a fort at Bombay and five factories on the west coast, Fort Marlborough and three factories in Sumatra, and factories in China, Persia and on the Red Sea. St. Helena was 'strongly fortified, and wholly possessed by us'.

The English (now the British) were increasingly in conflict with the French who, from their headquarters at Pondicherry, were gaining the support of Indian rulers, for both military help and trading concessions. By the 1740s the French, under Joseph François Dupleix, the Governor of Pondicherry, were encroaching on British territory. At first the French were successful. In 1748 Madras was besieged by the French fleet and captured on 10 September. But Dupleix was forced to return the city by the Peace of Aix-la-Chapelle in 1746. Fighting continued in India, and, from 1749, Clive[2] became the dominant figure. His lifting of the Siege of Arcot in 1751 made a deep impression on the Indians, and the French began to lose their influence. Suruj-ud-Daulah, the ruler of Bengal, sided with the French, and attacked Calcutta in 1756. The outnumbered garrison was forced to surrender.[3] Clive was sent to Bengal as Commander-in-Chief. His victory at the decisive Battle of Plassey (Placis Grove) in June 1757 ensured that the Company became the effective ruler of Bengal.

Fighting continued in other areas. In 1758 Fort St. George was again besieged by sea. One of the French ships came in close and bombarded ships near the Fort, but there was no reply from the land for an hour because the keys to the ammunition had been mislaid. In August 1759 a Dutch fleet from Batavia attacked Calcutta but was heavily defeated, ending Dutch power in India; in 1799 their company went bankrupt. There were repeated French defeats and in January 1761 Pondicherry surrendered. The Treaty of Paris (1752) ended all French military activity; their trading company collapsed in 1769. The rulers of Bengal and Oudh, rebelling against the Emperor, were defeated by the British at the Battle of Buxar (1764). This brought the Emperor under the protection of the Company which acquired free trading rights over large tracts of territory and a huge income. But to guard its reputation in Europe the Company took care to make it clear that this was all done on the authority of the Emperor.

For the war with the French the Company had formed its own regular armies, for which it recruited Indians, in the three Presidencies (Bengal, Madras, Bombay) each with its own medical service. These were now reinforced by Royal troops and ships. The first King's regiment reached India in 1760 bringing with it the first officers of the Army Medical Department. With the arrival of the extra soldiers there was a steady increase in the populations of Fort St. George and Calcutta. The British began to see themselves as living in cities rather than trading posts, although there was only a small increase in the number of civilians, whose entry to India was strictly controlled by the Company. Women were now allowed to come out to India but there was still a great shortage. In 1700 the population of Madras was 300,000; there were 400 English – 114 civilians including 19 women, and the rest soldiers. They all tried to make life as much like 'home' as possible, and they began to distance themselves from Indians and from some of the Indian customs that they had adopted earlier. The King's soldiers, not involved in trade, regarded themselves as socially superior to the Company's men. Their officers were given precedence over the Company's officers, and the rivalry between them sometimes interfered with military action; this was not resolved until the reforms of 1788 (p. 147). They had no interest in India or Indians, and their arrogance was part of the growing contempt by the British generally.

The Company's senior officials were living in great state. In Madras the Governor never went out except in procession, with two servants to drive away the flies. Official duties might not be very arduous. Mr Cunningham, the Head of a factory, who was bred a Surgeon, and had turned Virtuoso, would spend whole Days in contemplating on the Nature, Shape, and Qualities of a Butterfly or a Shellfish, and left the Management of the Company's Business to others as little capable as himself.

The Directors were still urging just behaviour towards Indians but the British were becoming increasingly overbearing. Physical abuse was common and was tolerated in a way that would have been impossible in earlier times when Company authority was stronger. The British continued to favour the Muslims. Hindus were slothful and, in the wealthier classes, deliberately fat, since fatness was a sign of wealth and status.

> The Asiatics in general prefer a sedentary life, and are surprised to see a European walk for exercise or pleasure; much more so to behold the English ladies and gentle-men take the trouble of dancing themselves, when they can have a variety of dancers and singers for money.

The British, active even in the heat, attributed much of the disease among the Hindus to their habits. The brahmins were not seen in their role as ministers and administrators but only as 'priests and mendicants with an unintelligible philosophy'. Contact with Hindu traders gave rise to the idea of the 'gentle Hindu', for the banyans were by nature inoffensive. If they quarrelled they never went beyond the 'Tongue-tempest or Banian Fight'. There were many complaints about their sharp practices but they were also capable of 'great probity and fidelity'. One sect of Hindus, the Mahrattas, were fierce warriors who caused the British endless trouble until they were finally subdued in the war of 1805 (p. 185).

Communication was still hindered by problems with language. Hindus and Muslims had Persian in common which 'all in India of distinction speak'. Most of the British did not take the trouble to learn more of an Indian language than that needed to give orders to their servants. All business was still conducted in pidgin Portuguese or through an interpreter. In their schools Indians only learned their mother tongue so that they were unable to speak English. The brahmins never studied any European language.

The strict rules of Hindu hygiene made social intercourse difficult.[4] But in Bombay there was also the Parsee community with very different customs. They were excellent shipbuilders, and came to control the Company's shipyard. It was permissible to dine with them and set up business partnerships. Cross-entertaining was mostly with Muslim nobles and princes who were interested in European habits and artefacts. There was increasing contempt for 'the servant-class in the Presidency towns', particularly by the King's soldiers. But every European had to have a Hindu banyan if he was trading or had troops to pay. These agents were generally regarded as 'deceitful, tedious, and rich (lending to their masters at 10 per cent)'.

The caste-system meant that every household had to have a large number of servants, who all 'conspired to keep the numbers up and to increase their wages as their master rose in the world'. The answer to complaints about this was that it was an 'all time custom'. One Indian custom that the British adopted was the hookah (p. 250). A special servant, the houccaburdar, was needed to tend this and to charge the bowl with its mixture of tobacco and spices. Hookahs came into fashion from about 1728, and by the 1760s were almost universal for women as well as men. The highest compliment that a woman could pay to a man was for her to smoke his hookah (after the mouthpiece had been changed). The regular dose was two-three charges after each of four meals, and the servant accompanied his master when he went out to dinner.

There was no contact with higher-class Indian women. In Vedic times women were able to hold high positions and to take part in religious ceremonies. With the rise of Hinduism they began to lose their freedom. Purdah[5] was brought to India by the Muslims and was adopted by some high-caste Hindus to protect their women from the invaders. Purdah among Muslim women was so strict that even if the house caught fire they would not leave the zenana[6] but would rather die there with their children. The seclusion of purdah meant that many women were poorly educated, with a monotonous existence and no exercise. Anaemia and bone diseases were common, leading to complications in childbirth. They were not allowed to receive any male medical contact except to have their pulse felt through a hole in the curtain. The Hindu physician made his diagnosis from the woman's handkerchief which she had rubbed all over her body to moisten it with her sweat:

> this handcercher the physitian puts into a bason of faire
> water and steepes it, and by the smell of the water knowes
> the distemper.

A high-caste woman giving birth was supervised entirely by the dais, old women of the *chumar*[7] caste, who prescribed for all female complaints, and were expert at procuring abortions. Hindu women were allowed to show themselves but they were always accompanied, and they were thus as well-protected as 'the impenetrable Moors'. The British were asked how they could allow their wives to talk to other men. When they said that they relied on their virtue, they were told that 'if butter is trusted too near the fire, it will hardly keep from melting'.

The early traders had sensibly modified their clothing to suit the climate. But this was now out of favour, and the high style of living demanded full European dress. The soldiers had always insisted on regulation uniforms, even though it was realized that the regimental dress of wool with a black hat was quite 'improper' for a hot climate. Apoplexy was a common consequence, and needed urgent bleeding if death was to be avoided (p. 106). The arrival of the King's soldiers led to the even stricter rule that uniforms should be worn in every detail as in Europe. It became a matter of military pride to take no notice of the heat – 'they wore heavy laced uniforms, curled and powdered wigs, skin-tight breeches and tight polished boots.' At official entertainments the ladies kept their 'stays and decorated heads as in Europe'. The men appeared in 'full dress, with bags[8] and swords', with the coat buttoned up to the throat. Judges in Court wore full robes and wigs, and changed their linen four times a day.

There were some concessions to the heat. Palanquins and umbrellas were seen as sensible precautions. But a palanquin cost 'not less than thirty pounds sterling a year', and this, together with the hire of a boy to carry the umbrella, was forbidden to the junior factors by the economical Company's edict of 1754. The Directors were warned that these young men had long distances to walk to transact the Company's business, and, for one newly arrived from England, it would be almost impossible to do this in the hot months 'without getting an inflammatory fever'.

One of the lesser afflictions of the newcomers was 'prickly heat' (*lichen tropicus*) in the hot months of June and July, described as

> a sharp pricking pain like the points of pins penetrating the body in every part, so that it is difficult to lie down in bed. It is, however, considered a sign of vigorous health. Newcomers are more subject to it than old residents, arising, as is supposed, from the superior richness or nicer susceptibility of the blood and general system.

Cold bathing often aggravated it but sailors seemed to spend a lot of time in the water, covered with pimples, without trouble. It was best to keep cool and quiet until acclimatized. If the sufferer could show 'stoical apathy' for the first few minutes of the attack 'the tiger will slink away for a time'.

But for the army on campaign, as often recorded by the surgeons, the heat could be lethal. The soldiers' tents, consisting of a single sheet of canvas, might have an inside temperature as high as 116°. Even in the officers' tents, which had a separate awning several feet above the canvas, the temperature would rise to 114°.

> Various Birds of the Forrest took shelter in the Tents, could not be driven out, and drank water when offered them as readily as if they had been brought up tame – a Hare came into the Tent of Adjutant Gee and drank water out of his hand ...
>
> The transition between health and fever, life and death, was so sudden that medicine had not time to operate, and our men died rapidly. On the march, with the sun high, the coup-de-soleil frequently struck the European soldiers with instant death.

Sudden death from heat-stroke (siriasis) was also common in inland stations:

> We have lost two Officers and Six Privates out of about 30 who have been taken ill of Fevers. Five of the Privates died from two to six hours after they first complained ... Some times the Men without any previous illness fell down Dead at Rollcalling ... many Pallanquin Boys died suddenly on the Roads ...

The disease took various forms, but one was particularly insidious:

> The Patient generally feels himself languid and faintish with slight headack and heat of Skin, and in this state generally lies down on his Cot without complaining much to them around him, his Comrades imagining him to be a Sleep, pay but little attention till they are disturbed by a croaking and noisy breathing and convulsive tremors and shaking over his legs and arms, by this time the Patient has lost the power of speech and deglutition, his face is livid ... there is a dreadful heat of skin which is like a burning coal ... the Patient seldom survives this Stage of the Disease above half an hour.

As the men began to realize the dangers, they reported as soon as they felt ill so that treatment was more successful. Treatment consisted of bleeding from the temporal artery (to reduce congestion of the brain without weakening the general system), cold compresses to the head after cutting the hair, cupping the back of the neck, and large doses of calomel. The medical officers were continually urging the authorities to move the troops regularly to healthier stations.

Up to the mid-eighteenth century the sickness-rate and mortality generally were still high, although there would then be a gradual improvement. 'The poor Factors and Writers have a hard bargain with the Company', but there was 'an Opportunity of growing rich sooner than at more healthful Places.' Up-country, diseases were not the only hazard. James Rennell,[9] on his surveying expeditions, was frequently laid up with fever, but was also involved in a skirmish which left him with four sabre wounds. It was six days before he got to a surgeon, and he was 'generally much troubled by tigers'.

Even the main Company settlements were still dangerously unhealthy. Bengal was the worst – in the ten years 1747-56, 74 per cent of the Company's servants died, and the overall mortality from 1707-75 was 57 per cent. The land surrounding Calcutta was 'an immense woody and jungly marsh' which was not cleared for fear of enemy attack. Woods and swamps were good natural defences but they were lethal to the defenders. In August 1720 there were 1,200 British; before the beginning of January there had been 450 registered burials. Even if the newcomers survived the 'salting' period, some of them suffered recurrent ill-health which would force them to return home. In the rainy season from June to October the country became a sheet of water. At high tide (twice in twenty-four hours) parts of Calcutta would be under four feet of water. Many Europeans drowned, but the natives swam well and escaped. Fort William was on the most unhealthy part of the river; 100-150 partially burned bodies floated every day past Diamond Harbour, the main anchorage of the Company's ships which might spend several months there.

> They entirely burn the bodies of the rich; but only disfigure those of the poor with the flames, and throw them into the river, where they float in great numbers, and are preyed on by the crows.

In an average year 300 sailors died – more than a quarter of the crews moored there. In the hot season the city was only kept clean by 'hungry jackals by night, and ravenous vultures, kites, and crows by day'. Company writers with urgent correspondence to deal with sat naked in large tubs into which cold water was poured by servants.

The East Indies were even more unhealthy. At Bantam, where the Dutch had added canals to make the city more like Europe, any small scratch would 'turn to a putrid ulcer down to the bone in twenty-four hours'. In June 1768 there were 5,490 Europeans in Batavia; 1,338 were in hospital, and 2,434 died in the following twelve months. Conditions were as bad in China and on the Persian Gulf where 'few of our factory escape putrid, intermitting fevers'; some of them recovered, but most died of 'obstructions of the liver'.

Bombay had been under siege (1687-90) in the war with the Emperor over the establishment in Bengal. This was followed by an epidemic that killed more men than the siege – only 60 were left out of 800. The corruption of the air in the monsoons was shown by the abundance and size of venomous creatures, with 'Toads as large as small Ducks'. But Bombay was now more wholesome than Calcutta. A wall had been built to keep out the sea to prevent it forming a marsh. Manuring the coconut trees with putrid fish was forbidden. Draining the marshes on the landward side started in 1721. The air was purer, but many Europeans still died there. Constitution seemed to have nothing to do with it – the strongest were often in most danger. Death could occur suddenly: 'we have known two instances of dining with a gentleman, and being invited to his burial before supper time.'

Madras was generally regarded as the healthiest of the three Presidencies. But Fort St. George was badly sited; it was rumoured that the only reason for such a choice was that the Governor had a mistress in nearby St. Thomas. The area round the Fort was infested with snakes and other vermin that were a danger to the inhabitants. The city was surrounded by stagnant swamps and ponds, which, like the beach on the other side,

> were covered at all hours of the day with natives, in the act of relieving nature from her burdens, to take advantage of the water for washing afterwards, which is their invariable custom.

In the city there was smoke and 'mosquitoes, rats, cockroaches, scorpions and bugs everywhere'. The smoke might give some relief from mosquitoes, but the windows had to be shut, and then there was no fresh air. The only cleaning of the sandy streets was by kites, crows, dogs and clouds of flies.

The Presidency Governments took little responsibility for public health.[10] The first rudimentary measures were in Calcutta, where J. Z. Holwell[11] in 1752 carried out the first census and, in 1755, made the first attempt to provide a clean water-supply. He gave a full description of the traditional Indian method of inoculation for smallpox (p. 91) in a report to the College of Physicians in London in 1767.

The Directors were now asking that the Bills of Mortality (p. 86) should include details of the 'Distempers of the Deceased', so that London physicians could advise suitable remedies, in case the surgeons in India were not skilled enough. But London had nothing much new to offer. There was now a general belief that the experimental methods of the seventeenth century did not improve the actual treatment of patients. A number of more speculative 'systems' were in vogue, such as the brunonian.[12] The scientific approach was not revived until the work of anatomists, physiologists and pathologists in the second half of the century. A university degree was required to become a Fellow of the Royal College of Physicians, but physicians provided only a very small part of the general medical care. Most of the patients were treated by surgeon-apothecaries who were still trained by apprenticeship. All practitioners were always in competition with numerous quacks. Folk-medicine was popular with all classes, and the gentry were as likely to take the advice of the quack as of the physician. Lunatics were still thought to be under the influence of supernatural forces and therefore incurable; this did not change until madness began to be seen as a 'disease' in the second half of the century. There were some advances in obstetrics but infant mortality remained very high: one in five infants died in their first year; one in three died before the age of five. Overall life-expectancy was about thirty-five years. There had been a start on measures to control smallpox. From the early years of the century the Royal Society had been discussing inoculation which had long been known and practised in Turkey, India (as reported by Holwell (p.108), and China. Spurred by Lady Mary Wortley Montagu's experiences of the good results of *ingrafting* in Constantinople in 1717, inoculations were carried out in England from the 1720s, and the numbers increased rapidly in the epidemics of the 1740s and 50s.

British surgeons in India, in spite of the doubts of the Directors, now felt that they had the experience of Indian diseases that allowed them to prescribe with confidence. There might be debate in England about the place of Peruvian bark in the treatment of fevers but all surgeons in the East agreed that it was not only the best cure but the best way to prevent recurrence. All ships, particularly those heading up river in Bengal, were advised to take large quantities of bark, even leaving other drugs behind, 'as bark is procured there with great expence and difficulty'. In Europe, bleeding was still 'the principal remedy in the cure of all inflammatory diseases'. Company surgeons at first had routinely bled the men on the outward voyage as a preventive measure. But they had abandoned this when they found that it made no difference to the incidence of disease. In India all surgeons were becoming more conservative, especially in fevers, where bleeding was seen to cause further weakness and exacerbation of the fever. They agreed that Europeans, on arrival in the tropics, 'bear evacuations much better than afterwards'. Sailors, too, with their intemperance and excesses, needed and withstood bleeding better than landsmen. But it was quite different after a long stay in a hot climate, and when treating Indians they had found that bleeding should be carried out with even greater caution. Dysentery in India, in contrast to Europe, was so resistant to treatment that only mercury would do any good. This had to be given with care as it was easy to overdose, and patients with scurvy were especially vulnerable. But many cases did well with careful mercurialization combined with opium. Ipececuanha was effective in some cases. In hepatitis, again in contrast to European opinion, the efficacy of mercury had been established; it gave the best chance of preventing an abscess in the liver, which was almost invariably fatal (p. 90).

The attempts to increase immunity to Indian diseases by 'indianization' had been abandoned when the bad results of the Portuguese regime were seen (p. 68). But some surgeons thought that a diet of Indian food might be a factor in increasing resistance. It was recognized that a heavy European diet was not the way to preserve health in the tropics. But the vegetarian diet of the Hindus was not sustaining enough – 'it softens and effeminates so that they are not capable of a strong and manly exertion of their reason.'

The debate was carried over to the healing of wounds. Since there was no longer any need to keep a wound open to let out the 'bad humours' (p.23), the aim was 'healing by first intention' by stitching the edges together. Most surgeons thought that a European diet was essential for quick healing. But there were still a number of reports which suggested the opposite – 'the wounds of those used to a vegetable diet, are much sooner and easier cured than those of such as eat flesh.' It was agreed that the European soldier withstood loss of blood better than the Indian, and this was attributed to his meat diet. But he was just as liable to infection and delayed healing of his wounds. Some Indians were cured of wounds that would be mortal in a European, 'and that with little more than binding the wound together, to the astonishment of the English surgeons'. The higher castes were

> cured by their own people that follow the camp, who dress their wounds with the extract of herbs: in short, they are almost self-cured. Many wounds, which in an European would make an amputation necessary, can in them be cured without.

The increasing numbers of troops arriving in India were now more carefully 'seasoned' and allowed to acclimatize slowly, sometimes by keeping them in the ships off shore for a few months. The problem was that they were often urgently needed in the field. Mortality was always highest in the new arrivals. But if a man could survive the first few years, he might continue for many years in reasonable health.[13] Even the mosquitos didn't disturb their old Acquaintance half so much as the new ones who were spotted like the Small-pox by morning, while others of longer standing, had not a mark, even if in the same room and cot.

Some men, long resident in the East and well-seasoned, dreaded going home for fear of what they might suffer by another change of climate.

European women in India seemed to be more resistant than men to the 'endemic and popular diseases', and they were thought to have some special immunity. But, as Mrs Kindersley wrote from Madras in 1765:

> It is frequently said, though very unjustly, that this climate never kills the English ladies; and indeed, it must be allowed, that women do not so often die of violent fevers as men, which is no wonder, as we live more temperately, and expose ourselves less in the heat of the day; and perhaps, the tenderness of our constitutions sometimes prevents the violence of the disorder, and occasions a lingering, instead of a sudden, death. But most English women labor under the oppression of weak nerves, slow fevers, and bile ... these disorders, and the continual perspiration, soon destroy the roses on the cheeks of the young and beautiful, and gives them a pale yellow complexion.

The British surgeons were now more confident in their management of the common Indian diseases, using more European drugs but also some well-tried Indian preparations. Their patients would take Indian prescriptions but they rarely accepted treatment from Indian practitioners. There was, in general, a very low opinion of Indian Medicine at this time. The art of prognosis was an important part of classical Indian Medicine, but

> a Brachman being sent for to an English Gentlewoman, then labouring under a chronical Distemper, ask'd for her Water, and pouring some into a China Dish, let fall into it a Drop of Oil, declaring, that if the Oil sunk to the Bottom, it inevitably betoken'd Death, the spreading of it on the Urine, an Increase of the Distemper, and its swimming closely united, an Abatement.

The surgeons thought that

> the skill of their physical people is very mean ... they have a number of leaves, plants, barks, roots which they use in decoctions ... if one root, leaf, or herb fails, they put in others of different sorts. In fevers, they used pepper, and such-like inflammatory substances.

Their text-book

> was an account of the anatomy of man, who was said to be made up of two or three hundred thousand parts, ten thousand veins etc. And all this was laid down without form or order, either of history, disease or treatment.
>
> ... they never study, but, like the other casts, the son of a doctor is a doctor also, and so he will continue to be from generation to generation.

The Hindus in Surat

> have 85 different sects among them, that do not eat with one another ... Another sort of them are Doctors of Physick, who pretend to do great Cures by Amulets, Philtres and Prayers. They have some Skill in Simples and Minerals, which make them in great Esteem; but when their Skill in Physick produces not the promised Effects, then they persuade the Patient, that they ly under the Displeasure of some angry Deity, who must be appeased by Oblations and Penances, and when that Trick fails, they leave their Patients to work out their own Salvation.

Venereal diseases were treated with China Root only. 'All their medicines are of the cooler Sort, because of the Heat of the Country.' But all swellings were usually treated by the application of a hot iron. They had no hospitals, only the animal hospitals in the area round Surat (p. 55).

The Unani practitioners were no better:

> In Arabia ... we cannot expect to find great physicians. Those who there practise the art of medicine, know little more than the technical terms, such as they find them in the books of Avicenna, and some little matters about the use of simples.

Some Indians, particularly the rich and the nobles, were starting to prefer British doctors, and always when an operation was needed.

In the second half of the eighteenth century there was a gradual improvement in the sickness and mortality rates of the British in India. But this was probably due more to them changing some of their habits, and taking sensible precautions, than to any advances in medicine.[14] The changes started on the voyage where gross overcrowding had often led to the spread of infection. It was recognized that it was cheaper to keep soldiers and sailors in good health than to send out replacements. As the ships got larger and faster they could make more frequent calls to take in fresh meat, fruit and water, setting out again with 'three score hogs and a thousand fowls'. Turtles were a great delicacy that could be 'fed on almost two Months, without being weary', and ships would stop at Ascension specially to pick up a good supply. There were dolphins to catch, and one shark would provide a meal for the whole ship, but

> it was not much esteemed, except for the fins cooked in the Chinese fashion, which were one of those rare provocatives to venery that at once stimulate and strengthen.

There was less salt meat, and it could be 'counteracted' with sugar and tea. Every East Indiaman carried a baker, and fresh bread was also good against the salt; porter was used if there was no yeast. When the water became putrid, it was fermented with porter and sugar to make a 'brisk palatable small beer'. The ships were ventilated and fumigated, and the men as far as possible kept dry with stoves between decks and extra clothes from the slop chest. Large stocks of bark and ipecacuanha were carried to deal with the expected fevers. Scurvy was becoming less frequent, but there were still occasional outbreaks, and the connection with fresh fruit was not always made. Prudent captains would ensure that preventive measures started on the first day when the ship's stock of fresh vegetables and beer was finished, before the first signs of the disease:

> Every healthy seaman carries with him to sea a certain quantity or proportion of antiscorbutic humours. The stock may be preserved, if husbanded with care; but cannot, in that situation, be easily recovered, if once it is suffered to run down.

Putting scorbutic sailors on land meant that they would almost certainly be cured, but sometimes 'baffling winds, calms and currents' kept the ships out for several days, and the dead would then have to be 'committed to the deep, whom a few cocoa-nuts and tropical fruits might have preserved'.

By experiments at sea in May 1747 the Naval surgeon James Lind showed conclusively that scurvy was not due to the high level of salt in the air, and that 'oranges and lemons were the most effectual remedies for this distemper at sea'. He found it difficult to convince some of his contemporaries. Richard Mead, a prominent physician, continued to stress 'bad air' as the cause, and recommended a machine that he had invented to improve ventilation in ships. Publication of Lind's results made little immediate difference to the incidence of scurvy. The problem was the preservation of the active principle. Lind's method was to heat the juice to produce a 'rob' (syrup), or to mix it with rum.[15] Lemon juice was not issued officially to the Navy until 1795, and even later to the merchant service. West Indian limes were then introduced as cheaper, but they have less than half the vitamin C content of lemons. Since the recommended doses of lemon were barely sufficient, this was responsible for recurrent outbreaks of scurvy up to the middle of the nineteenth century.

While at sea, the health of the crew might remain good. It was not until

> arrival in Harbour, and after anchoring in sickly Places, that the men are attacked with the Diseases of the Country.

It was recognized that a ship anchored a short distance from land was protected against fevers. The dangerous tasks were landing to stock up with wood and water, especially after sunset, and, in the settlements, clearing the ground, especially in the rainy season. Natives could be paid to bring cargoes out to the ships. If landing was unavoidable the men should be back on board before sunset, and then kept off deck after sunset and before sunrise. Ports should be shut against the land breezes. The men were to smoke tobacco and the ship should be fumigated. The greatest risk was sleeping on shore. If this was essential, the men should take bark twice a day, and, for added protection, rinse their mouths with vinegar, and put small vinegar-soaked plugs in their nostrils. Neglect of these precautions 'had destroyed every year several thousand seamen'.

On land the natural history of 'malaria' was recognized, and precautions were known, if not always put into effect: the danger of marshes and wet soil, particularly in hot weather after the rainy season [leaving pools for the mosquito to breed]; remission in heavy rain and floods [washing away the breeding pools]; the protection afforded by a wood, so that cutting down the trees might be followed by an epidemic, and the protection of a large stretch of water [the mosquito has a range of two miles]. Some areas would always be recognized as unhealthy, and every factory should have a 'place of retreat', so that people could move there in the 'sickly seasons' – 'yet our factories abroad have never paid any attention to it.' Houses should be sited as high as possible above the dangerous marshy exhalations. Ventilation was essential, but doors and windows should not face a swamp. But Company officials were building grand two-storied town houses that were fiercely hot. The change was gradually made to 'more air and less light', with blinds, folding doors, 'tatties' (wet matting), punkahs (large swinging fans), and finally to lower ceilings and smaller windows. In the country the houses were usually of one storey – the bungalow[16] – both comfortable and cheap. These precautions would be helped by a regular intake of bark, and moderation in all things.

Over-eating, especially meat, was recognized as harmful in the heat, but, if required, freshly-killed meat should be collected at night immediately after killing, or it would not be fit to eat the next day. Some of the British came to relish the local food with its spices and variety, and might even prefer it to their cold-weather diet. They worried about the amount of fish that was served, but were cheered by the sight of the fishermen's villages, where there seemed to be more children than anywhere else, showing that a fish-diet 'was not a mortification and aid to continency'.

All water was suspect. The Ganges was still full of floating bodies and carrion, only partly dealt with by wild animals. Travellers carried their favourite supply with them; anything else was likely to cause 'many disorders, especially when not mixed with wine'. Foul water could be purified with powdered alum, or by filtering through gravel or sand.

Large quantities of alcohol were drunk by all classes, and even hardened European drinkers might find it difficult to keep up. But it was agreed that a moderate intake of wine was essential for health; claret was the best for preventing disease. Ladies should take one bottle a day, and gentlemen four or five. Casks of wine were always provided for the hospitals. Arrack,[17] the country spirit, was often impure, stronger than brandy, and 'very pernicious, especially to Europeans'.

Tea and coffee were now being drunk in large quantities – 'Coffee in the Morning, and the Tea about Four in the Afternoon'. They were cheap, and reputed to have medicinal properties (p. 250). The Company tried to promote tea as an alternative to alcohol, but there was no enthusiasm for this.

The British had learned many of the measures for preserving health in the tropics, and these were now being brought together and published. One of the first was by James Lind (p. 114) who gave a general account (1768) of all the precautions necessary on land as well as at sea, with emphasis on the needs of the Navy. He hoped that these would become more widely recognized:

> it is one thing for subordinates who have to obey orders, but
> their ignorance is highly blameable in commanders in chief.

He held to the widespread belief that:

> in all Countries, Providence has wisely ordered a provision of the most proper Remedies for their peculiar and endemic diseases.

But in spite of this there were some patients for whom 'a Retreat to a more Northern climate is absolutely needful to recover their wonted Tone and Vigour'.

At about the same time (Sir) John Pringle published his advice (1769) for improving the health of the Army on land in Europe. He urged greater cleanliness in general, and particularly in hospitals, with greater use of antiseptics. He recognized land scurvy (p.32) and recommended a diet with less salt meat and more fruit and vegetables. The hardships of a soldier's life demanded something stronger than water, and

> if some actually fall ill after hard drinking, it is certain a far greater number are preserved by taking these liquors in moderation.

For the Company, John Clark MD of Edinburgh wrote his *Observations* (1773) at the request of Sir John Silvester who 'presided over the medical concerns of the East-India Company'. Clark had been on two Company voyages, returning via China. He noted that the officers left the care of the health of the men to the doctors, and the doctors were foiled by the 'obstinacy and prejudices of the men', for:

> seamen and soldiers, as far as their health is concerned, can only be considered as adult children, who require authority to prevent them from doing themselves harm.

But the Company's ships had more space and less disease than the military transport where 'our ships of war so often resemble floating funerals; and our naval and military hospitals pest-houses'. He recorded all the diseases at sea and on land, with their remedies and the now more generally recognized rules for healthy living in the tropics. He urged the medical journals to help by publishing unsuccessful cases, instead of the successes 'with which medical publications abound'. The Company should send regular case-reports to all its surgeons.

This published information was put into effect by the better-trained practitioners who were being recruited by the Company – many of them graduates of the new medical schools. In London between 1720-45 five large teaching hospitals were founded. The Barbers and Surgeons had separated when The Corporation of Surgeons of London was formed in 1745. The Corporation gave certificates for posts in the Navy and Army, and in an Indiaman or as Assistant Surgeon to an Indian Presidency. In addition, the Company set up its own examining Board in London, and there were examinations in India for promotion and for local applicants. These examinations were not open to Indians. The Edinburgh University Medical School, founded in 1726, gave a broad training in both medicine and surgery which made its graduates particularly suitable for military, naval and Company service. By the middle of the century many of the Company surgeons were from Scotland. The new surgeons were often needed at once on active service, as in the war with the French from the 1740s. But after 1762 all Assistant Surgeons on arrival in India were appointed for at least three months to one of the General Hospitals.

These had been improved and enlarged to accommodate patients not directly employed by the Company. But they always had to give way to the needs of the military. In Madras the hospital was taken over in 1754 as it was needed as a barracks. Twelve houses were converted into a temporary hospital but this left the sick dangerously exposed. In 1757 the hospital was enlarged to accommodate 200-250 men. But as it was sited on high ground for medical reasons, it was badly placed in case of a siege, and orders were given for it to be demolished. Many of the sick then had no other protection than open straw sheds which became puddles with every heavy shower. In 1772 these were replaced by the solid building that is still part of the present-day General Hospital. The hospital in Calcutta was destroyed in the capture of the city in 1756 (p. 101). The rebuilt hospital, with additions, lasted until 1902. In Bombay the original hospital was replaced in 1733 and there was a separate hospital for the Navy. All unmarried soldiers were required to go to the hospital when they were sick, and a sentry was posted to stop them leaving before they were seen by the surgeon. Muster Rolls included the soldiers sent into hospital, their diseases and the dates of entry and discharge or death. The surgeons now had assistants, and there was a Steward to look after the feeding and clothing of the patients and special diets ordered by the surgeon. There was as yet no separate accommodation for the insane who were shipped home as soon as possible. The Indian treatment was to put the patients in

> a close Room, just big enough to hold them, and almost smoke them to death with Musk and cold Smells, which soon brings their brains into their right temperature, and so recovers them.

The hospitals were still for Europeans only. There were no hospitals for Indian civilians until the first (in Calcutta) in 1792. The first hospital for the Company's Indian troops, the sepoys,[18] was opened in 1760. Before this, when large numbers of sick were expected from the army on campaign, small garrison hospitals were prepared, where they were looked after by their own surgeons.

The medical training of Indians was continued in the General Hospitals. Competent dressers and compounders (p. 86) were given a certificate of proficiency by the Surgeon-in-charge. Their names would then be added to the payroll and they became eligible for pensions on the same terms as other Company employees. In 1738, in Bombay, the pay scales included Apothecary, Black Assistant and Black Doctor.

Diet in the hospitals was standardized at an allowance of beef or mutton up to one lb. per day, and two lbs. of bread, with arrack, wine and milk, 'increased according to the Nature of the Complaint'. The surgeon could order special diets for serious cases. The diet for sepoys was the same for all complaints: 'rice, doll [dahl – split pulse], ghee [boiled butter], and dried or salted Mumbaloes [bummelo – small fish], with some curry stuff', and 'wine and arrack occasionally if complaints require and Religion allows'. The average daily expense for a European in hospital was twice as much as for a sepoy. The men were charged for their food according to their rank: in 1713 a soldier paid four annas a day, a corporal six, and a sergeant half a rupee.[19] At first the soldiers paid nothing for their medicines. Later a charge was made, which was higher for venereal disease, in the hope that this would act as a deterrent. The sailors' expenses for their treatment were reclaimed from the captain of the ship. This sometimes led to treatment being cut short, as the captain economized by removing his crew from the hospital ahead of time.

From 1764 the surgeons contracted to supply everything necessary for the hospitals. This 'hospital contract' was given to the Senior Surgeons who were paid 18 rupees p.a. for each man in hospital. Out of this they had to pay for everything except clothing, European medicines, and the soldier's daily diet. These contracts were very lucrative as the holder could make a profit on the supply of drugs. They were hotly competed for, and some surgeons made large fortunes. There were complaints that the surgeons were encouraging men to plead sickness and stay in hospital longer than necessary. The system was abolished in 1815. The Directors were always concerned to save money, and they continually grumbled at the cost of the increasing number of hospitals. When the new hospital in Madras was proving too expensive, the surgeons were ordered to take charge alternately every six months to see whether they could rival one another in economies 'to recommend themselves'.

Surgeons were responsible for making the forecast of drugs and instruments needed, which had to be prepared eighteen months in advance for transmission to London. When the Directors complained that the indents for instruments were unnecessarily high, the surgeons pointed out that the fault lay in 'the Nature of this air, whose saltness subjects them very much to rust'. They relied on supplies of drugs from England but these were often damaged in storms or spoiled by spillage. There were frequent requests for greater care in the packing of supplies in London.

There were also complaints of deficiencies, particularly the short supply of essential drugs that could not be provided in India, such as bark and cantharides.[20] Some of the drugs were of poor quality when first supplied, and the Directors were repeatedly told that some of the medicines from London were useless. Others went bad in store or were destroyed by white ants. Stocks might be adequate at the centre but severe epidemics in outlying stations could produce shortages, and there were urgent requests for fresh supplies. Stocks were also reduced by destruction or capture in war. When medicines in the Public Store were exhausted, permission was given to buy them locally. But some of the country medicines were more suited to garrison practice. On field service there might be little need for them and they were often bulky to transport.

Surgical instruments and equipment were all sent out from England, and there were complaints of the quality. There were no arrangements for the repair of instruments, which had to be sent back to London, and their return was always slow. There were requests by the surgeons for a repair service to be set up locally with local craftsmen who had always been very skilled at producing high quality instruments (p. 9).

European medicines also reached India by private transactions or carried by individuals. Most of these were used in private practice. When central supplies ran out, grudging permission was given to buy from these private stocks. But there was a danger that the private supply of drugs would result in 'considerable private emolument', and this was against the best interests of the Company. 'All irregular practitioners and vendors of medicines' were required to have a licence from the Medical Board. Any servants of the Company who wished to deal in this way should leave the Company's service and 'obtain the permission of Government to settle in the country as private adventurers'. However, the European population in India was increasing rapidly, and many of them had no claim on the Company, which was their only source of 'wholesome drugs'. Control of all vendors of European medicines would save the Company money and would 'increase the demand for European medicines to an object of Commercial importance'. It would also encourage Indians to use this service, and 'introduce into India the knowledge of European Pharmacy'.

There was still no organized treatment of Indian civilians. But there were continual pleas from the very poor for medical help. Doctors travelling overland were advised to conceal all medical knowledge, or their lodgings would be overrun from morning to night. Higher caste Hindus would not usually seek treatment from a European, and would refuse it if offered, although there might be no suitable Indian remedy. Requests from the local (Muslim) rulers, often when a surgical operation was needed, continued throughout the eighteenth century. The Company was always ready to send out physicians and surgeons, and also to receive important patients if they came into the cities seeking medical advice. Medicines made good presents and could be used to bribe marauding bands when they came too close.

The first Indians to be treated in any number were the sepoys. They were mostly high-caste Hindus with a reputation for good discipline. They had first been recruited in Bombay (1677) and Madras (1686) where they were looked after by their own practitioners. Their numbers increased rapidly through the eighteenth century with the widespread fighting and the formal establishment of a Company army in each of the three Presidencies. Company surgeons now became responsible for their health; they sometimes found it difficult to distinguish genuine disease from symptoms produced by fear and emotion, as with cases of snake-bite (p. 95). The sepoys made excellent soldiers but their rigid caste-rules posed continuing problems for their medical officers (p. 121). The Hindu's fatalism was also a powerful factor. Ananda Ranga Pillai[21] recorded in his diary the illness of one of his relatives, who

> contracted venereal disease, which was complicated by an attack of diarrhoea ... in spite of the best medical advice available, succumbed to the attack ... since he was destined to live only so long.

This not only influenced the sepoy's response to treatment but his willingness to report early for medical attention.

Indian dressers were employed for attachment to each Native Regiment. The high-caste sepoys were forbidden by their rules to accept food or drugs that had been handled by a European or by one of another caste. Each battalion, therefore, had to have an Indian practitioner of the same caste to prepare and administer the drugs prescribed by the European medical officer. These 'doctors'[22] also acted as dressers for the wounded and at operations. In 1785 individual Battalion Hospitals were set up for the sepoys, which they much preferred to the General Hospitals. Surgeons to Native Regiments regarded these small hospitals as more necessary for Indians than for Europeans. There was the problem of getting the high castes to take food from any but their own caste. It was necessary for the families of the sick to come in and help, but no respectable woman would go to the General Hospital, and the Sepoy of Cast, holds the Hospital in abhorrence, and would rather submit to any hardship, or conceal the most dangerous distemper, than enter within its Walls.

The caste rules gave rise to other problems. Articles of diet, and their preparation, were very carefully specified, and high-caste Hindus would, and often did, starve on campaign, if their accustomed food could not be provided.[23] Travel overseas was also a sin to the orthodox, and this led to mutiny later (p. 210). But even if they could be forced on a sea-voyage, the sepoys would refuse to eat when their own provisions were exhausted and all that was left was salt beef. When they were ill they would often refuse to take the prescribed diet, and could not be persuaded that it might help their disease. There were similar problems later with vaccination (p. 177). The lower castes had no such scruples. While the sepoys would get ulcers and other disorders by refusing the necessary diet, convicts in the jails put on weight. Alcohol, highly regarded by the British for its medicinal properties, was prescribed in controlled doses for many complaints. While European troops would take this medicine readily enough, it was totally forbidden to the orthodox Hindu.

British surgeons continued to treat noblemen and their families. Muslims favoured their own practitioners but every princely house had both hakeems and vaidyas on its staff, and the patients seem to have taken the prescriptions of either indiscriminately. As the Company relaxed its restrictions on visitors, European doctors, not in the pay of the Company, began to come out to India to make their fortunes. Many Indian courts had one or more European physicians and surgeons on their staff in addition to their European military advisers. In 1778 the Nawab of Arcot had eight European practitioners – two physicians and six surgeons of various nationalities – as well as a larger number of both Muslim and Hindu practitioners. One of his British physicians from 1787-1803 was Sir Paul Jodrell who had been appointed after a request from the Nawab direct to George III. Jodrell was upset to find himself in competition with all the other Europeans as well as the local experts. He was allowed to see patients outside the Court, and he often visited the town where he was in competition with Portuguese and French physicians. Many Indian rulers were obsessed by the fear of being poisoned. Their European doctors had to be at the beck and call of their employers, often for trivial complaints or simply to test their loyalty. The patient would often ask for, and take, the widely differing prescriptions of the three systems of medicine. The problems of treating high-born Indian women continued, with the physician only allowed to contact his patient by feeling her pulse through a hole in a curtain.

Private practice was first mentioned officially in 1764 but it had always been allowed. The Company insisted that any patient not in their employment should pay the doctor for his services. All the Company's servants were entitled to free treatment, except for venereal disease; some of them chose to be private patients. From them and wealthy Indians the surgeon could make a large income to supplement his meagre salary.

The salaries offered by the Company were still low,[24] but there was no difficulty in recruiting well-qualified young doctors, and the Directors resisted attempts in India to raise their salaries, writing in 1761:

> the surgeons that we send abroad to our Capital Settlements are always acquainted with this salary and emoluments and we find no difficulty in having able men of that profession as well as all other branches of our service. If their heads are turned, give us due notice, that we may call them home again and supply their places with men of more humble mind, though perhaps not inferior talents.

As well as private practice (which met with 'very liberal returns') there were other 'emoluments' for the surgeon – allowances, which usually considerably exceeded his salary, for housing, servants and household supplies. While serving in the field with the Army he was entitled, like all Company servants, to batta.[25] In the towns, to avoid undue exertion in the hot weather, he was given a 'Palankeen allowance' for his official visits. All Company servants could expect rich presents every year from the banyan brokers. The surgeons were included in this, and also in the President's bounty at Christmas.

Surgeons in private practice were notorious for the high fees they charged. Drugs were very expensive, and treatment often included bleeding and purging which always went together but were charged separately. One visit cost one gold mohur,[26] and the charge for one ounce of salts was one rupee, and for one ounce of bark three rupees. A complaint from Bombay that there was little or no private practice and that no surgeon had gone home with a fortune was met with the retort that this was because of the surgeons' extravagant living in India. In 1742 the Directors accused the surgeons of using drugs from the official store in their private practice, 'either in the cure of Venereal distempers or among the natives or other inhabitants, for which they are well paid'. They proposed to send one quarter of the medical supplies out separately for the surgeons to buy for their practice. The surgeons replied that the rate of venereal disease among the Company's servants was always so high that, when the allocation of medicines for them was finished, they should be allowed to use some of the supplies intended for private patients.

The Company had always tried to restrict the amount of private trading because it distracted its servants from their duty to make a profit for the Company. Throughout the seventeenth century the permitted amount was so small that the factors, who generally paid little attention to the edicts of their masters, could only make a profit out of illicit trading. Gradually a small amount of tonnage in locally-trading and homeward-going ships was set aside for private trading. This tonnage was gradually increased, the higher ranks having the greater share. It was then only bad luck that prevented the commander of a ship making a fortune, and the lower ranks pro rata. Company servants rented the ships waiting in harbour for the north-east monsoon for the voyage home. They used them for local trading along the coasts and made most of their profits this way while still maintaining the Company's monopoly of the home market.

Before 1764 there was no home leave. But for many in India at this time the aim was to make a quick fortune and return to England as a 'nabob'.[27] The rumours of fabulous wealth and the obvious success of the returning 'nabobs' encouraged others to make their way to India. But the Company always kept strict control of travellers; licences were required for residence. Surgeons arriving on private ships were compelled to return on the same ship. If they were found on shore without a Company licence they were sent home at once. If a serving surgeon wished to return to England, often because of ill-health, he had to resign from the service and apply for reappointment. To save the cost of the passage to England he would wait until there was a vacancy for a surgeon on an East Indiaman for the homeward voyage.

For the war with the French most of the Company's medical officers were military surgeons. They were kept very busy and became very experienced. They were therefore considered first for promotion to all important posts. The fewer civilian surgeons had less to do.[28] As there were no hospitals or dispensaries for Indian civilians their practice might be limited to the few Company servants at a peripheral station and there was little private practice. This meant that they had time for business and trading activities. Some abandoned their profession to concentrate on local industries and land speculation. Some would stay on as Assistant Surgeons in civil posts in the hopes of the next vacancy for Full Surgeon, but this might take twenty years. The difference in pay was not very great and it might not be enough to compensate them for moving from the *mofussil* (the country stations) where they were profitably engaged in some commercial activity such as the indigo trade. If they were criticized for their involvement in trade, they replied that they were bringing the benefits of new industries to the local people. But whatever their duties they all counted as civilians so that, when the King's troops arrived in 1760, a Chief Surgeon of many years experience in India came lower in the scale than the most junior subaltern out from England (p.147).

Physicians might still try to assert their superiority over surgeons. In 1778 Dr Jackson, a physician from London, made his way independently to Calcutta and incensed the surgeons there by applying to be made Inspector of all the Company's hospitals, on the grounds that, as he was a physician, he should have priority over all the other medical officers who were only surgeons.

In 1764, as part of the reorganization of the Bengal Army following the war with the French, all Company medical officers in Bengal were incorporated to form the Bengal Medical Service.[29] The other two Presidencies, Madras and Bombay, soon followed the same pattern. All medical officers then became primarily military surgeons for the regular troops of the Company's armies.[30] They were only temporarily lent for civil duties, in which they formed a reserve for the army and were liable for recall at any time. This pattern continued until the disbandment of the Indian Medical Service in 1947

Notes

1 There were swellings in the groin, which may have been a hydrocele (fluid round the testicle) or possibly venereal disease, and 'a violent pain in his posteriors'.

2 Robert Clive (1724-74) had arrived in Madras as a Company writer in 1744.

3 'The Black Hole of Calcutta'. In his account, J. Z. Holwell (f.n.11) stated that he was one of 23 survivors of the 146 who were imprisoned on the night of 20 June 1756. Released the next day, but still a prisoner in irons and covered with boils, he knew that over-eating after starvation would be fatal: 'our rice-and-water diet, designed as a grievance to us, was certainly our preservation, for, could we (circumstanced as we were) have indulged in flesh and wine, we had died beyond all doubt.'

4 To take water from a Hindu, the European had to tilt his head back for the water to be poured into his mouth so as not to 'defile by hands or lips'. One man borrowed a flute from a Hindu; when he returned it, it was at once thrown in the river.

5 *parda*, curtain (Pers.).

6 *zan*, woman (Pers).

7 leather-workers, a very low caste.

8 wigs with the back hair enclosed in a bag.

9 The first Surveyor-General of India.

10 All major legislation came in the second half of the nineteenth century.

11 John Zephaniah Holwell had come out as a Company surgeon in 1732. He survived the Black Hole of Calcutta (1756), and finally became Governor-General of Bengal. He was appointed FRS in 1767, the second Company medical officer after John Fryer.

12 John Brown (1735-88) – all disease is due to excess or lack of stimulus, and is therefore to be treated by depletion or stimulation. This is similar to Ayurveda, with depletion by purges, enemas and bleeding.

13 Dr James Anderson made one voyage as surgeon in a Company ship in 1759, and again in 1761 when he landed. He had a very distinguished career, serving continuously in India until his death in 1810 at the age of 72.

14 Just as improvements in Britain in the second half of the nineteenth century were due more to sanitary and public health measures than to medical treatment.

15 Even when freshly made in this way, the vitamin C content is reduced by 50 per cent, and further on storage. This was not solved until the development of canning in the nineteenth century.

16 *bangla*, of Bengal (Hindi).

17 At Fort St. George the Company had the sole power to make an inferior, very strong brew which they sold to Indians. The Company also had the monopoly of tobacco and betel (p. 244), and made large profits on all three.

18 *sipahi*, soldier (Pers).

19 sixteen annas = one rupee = c. 2s.

20 Preparations of Spanish Fly, *Cantharis vesicatoria*, 'the most powerful medicine in the materia medica', used for blistering. A patient with paralysis might be blistered from the back of his head to the base of his spine.

21 The 'Indian Pepys', *dubash* (broker/interpreter) to Dupleix when he was Governor of Pondicherry in the second quarter of the eighteenth century.

22 In the Madras Army they were known officially as 'Black Doctors'.

23 A similar problem occurred in W.W.II when a battalion of an Indian infantry regiment had to be withdrawn from active service in Burma with severe nutritional deficiency.

24 In 1757 annual salaries were: Governor £200, chaplain £50, senior merchant £40, surgeon £36, junior merchant £30, factor £15, writer £5.

25 *bhata*, an extra allowance (Hindi).

26 one mohur = 16 rupees; one rupee = c. 2s.

27 *nawab*, a deputy (Hind.). In India, a title of rank without any office attached. Applied in England, in the eighteenth century, to anyone returning from India with a fortune.

28 This changed by the middle of the nineteenth century when the civil surgeon was over-worked and the military surgeon had time for research (p. 216).

29 The formation of the Bengal Medical Service is taken as the date of origin of the Indian Medical Service.

30 In 1749 there were 29 surgeons in India; in 1785 there were more than 230.

Chapter Nine
The end of the Mogul Empire

With the Emperor under the 'protection' of the British from 1764 (p. 102) the loss of central authority and of control by local rulers allowed increasing extortion from the people by Indian officials and money-lenders – 'extortion was not unknown before, but now it was doubled or quadrupled'. The Indian agents of the Company were deeply involved. The Company was still trading through Hindu banyans who were all closely linked and ran all the business. Even when the Company officials, who could not speak Bengali, decided to employ their own agents, they were unable to choose the best and most honest. But many of the officials behaved as badly as their agents. With no control from Calcutta over private trading, Company officials were able to divert the main local monopolies of salt, betel and tobacco in particular. Bengal was also overrun by illegal traders and adventurers – 'European vagabonds' – determined to make a fortune as quickly as possible and get home before tha climate killed them.[1] There were marauding groups of bandits, and the police were ineffective. The judicial courts were open to bribery by wealthy Indians, and prisoners were treated unjustly.[2]

In 1763 the Directors re-appointed Clive who had left India in 1760. By April 1765 he was back in Madras. He instituted the regular collection of taxes, and was able to reduce the level of corruption in Bengal before he went home in 1767. His military operations gained further political power for the Company over a wide area. He had obtained from the Emperor a grant of land between Calcutta and Madras which would link up the Company's possessions. The local ruler objected and, joining with Haider Ali, the ruler of Mysore, threatened Madras. They were defeated by Company forces, and a treaty in April 1769 ended the First Mysore War. But the Company was continually engaged in wars in other parts of the country. The Rajah of Tanjore was regarded as a dangerous power in the Carnatic. In September 1773 a Company force captured Tanjore, and took the Rajah and his family prisoner. Haider Ali attacked again in 1780 with a large army with French officers, and gained three major victories. He died in 1782, but the Second Mysore War was continued by his son, Tippoo, who was finally defeated and peace signed in 1784.

Bengal, temporarily free of military activity, was now devastated by famine. The civil adminstration was still under Indian officials of the Central Government when 'The Bengal Famine' broke out in 1770.[3] There had been partial failure of the crops the year before, but the authorities who were responsible for relief had continued rigorously to enforce the land-tax while laying in extra supplies for the troops. In the early part of 1770 disease broke out and by May more than one-third of the population in the worst-affected areas had died.

> The husbandmen sold their cattle; they sold their implements of agriculture; they devoured their seed-grain; they sold their sons and daughters, till at length no buyer of children could be found ... Day and night a torrent of famished and disease-stricken wretches poured into the great cities ... The streets were blocked up with promiscuous heaps of the dying and the dead ... even the dogs and the jackals, the public scavengers of the East, became unable to accomplish their revolting work.

In spite of urgent representations, Central Government failed to realize the extent of the disaster and continued to insist on full levy of the land-tax, even increasing it by 10 per cent in April 1770 for the following year. There were no effective relief measures. Attempts to prevent the hoarding and export of grain for private profit were frustrated by corruption at all levels of the administration. Lack of transport meant that little could be done to bring in relief supplies, even if there had been the organization to set this up. Although there were good crops the next year there were too few people left to harvest them. In nine months ten million had died. Large areas were left deserted, and reverted to jungle. The effects were felt for the next forty years.

The British had no direct responsibility for relief measures. Troops were moved out of affected areas but as they were simply marched from one famine area to another they consumed the local supplies wherever they went. There were no subscription-lists and no restrictions on the export of grain as there would be in famines in the nineteenth century (p. 223).

Many of the British at this time had little contact with Indians, and were not concerned with their welfare. The only connection might be in business, competing with crafty merchants, or adminstering justice to criminals in courts corrupted by bribery. The old Indian governing classes were retreating into seclusion, leaving the lower classes to represent Indians to the British. Their view of the Indian character was also influenced by missionaries who worked mostly with the lowest classes — the pariahs. For some of the British the only contact was with their servants, and they only learned enough of the local language to give them instructions.

To conform with caste rules, large numbers of servants were needed — each caste would only carry out one very specific task. A captain in garrison needed 30 servants, and, in the field, 30 porters. On campaign, an army of 103 officers and 6,624 troops needed 19,729 servants, 12,000 market people and 19,000 cattle (an army on the march had to take all its food with it).

With Indian servants there was no problem with keeping food, for no Hindu would touch anything that had been touched by a European. They were careful about their own food; but the bobachee (male cook) was slovenly in the preparation of food for Europeans. Every gentleman was attended by his own servants when invited out, so that it was hard to keep cool with the crowd round the table. Most important was the aub-dar, responsible for cooling the water and the wine. Also required were a peruquier (when both men and women wore their hair 'full-dressed'), a tailor, a laundryman, a syce (groom) and a sirdar at the head of them all. Malays were much in demand as gardeners; they had a traditional skill with growing medicinal herbs and making up prescriptions. In spite of their numbers, the total expense was no more than in England. European servants were twelve times as expensive and needed nearly as many attendants as their masters. A palanquin was essential in the heat and when puddles prevented walking. At least seven bearers were needed; on long distances in good weather it was possible to cover 400 miles in five days.

The agents (dubash/banyan) gave rise to many complaints. In their roles as 'banker, purveyor, pimp and interpreter' they were able to cheat their masters who could not speak their language. The money-lenders were always liberal and civil to gentlemen, and would keep them from starving.

A contemporary[4] described 'A Day as is commonly spent by an Englishman in Bengal':

> He is called at eight, a lady quits his side, going to her own apartment or out of the compound ... he is dressed without any greater exertion than if he was a statue ... a barber shaves him, cuts his nails, cleans his ears ... he washes his hands and face, walks to breakfast of tea and toast ... attended by hair-dresser and huccabadar with hookah, he smokes and eats alternately ... banian with other attendants and solicitors until 10 ... palanquin with cavalcade of 8-12 in distinctive livery and 8 bearers ... visits until 2 ... a good dinner attended by his own servant and then the hookah ... at 4 he is undressed and sleeps until 7-8 ... then as at breakfast with the hair-dresser etc. A handsome coat for ceremonial visits until supper at 10. The company stay until 12-1 preserving great sobriety and decency ... he is conducted to his bedroom where he finds a female companion to amuse him until the hours of seven or

eight next morning ... with no greater exertions than these, do the Company's servants amass the most splendid fortunes.

The British now felt that Indians should treat all Europeans with respect at all times, so that to be stopped and searched by native customs officials was regarded as insolence. But they took care not to offend their soldiers who were brave and faithful but would rebel at anything that went against their religious beliefs. Since poultry were regarded as pollution by Hindus, any attempt to get them to wear a feather in their head-dress could lead to mutiny. When Muslim soldiers applied for leave for a feast, there was official guidance for the officers to decide whether, in granting the application, they were interfering with military duties, or, in refusing it, infringing the religious rights of the men.

The number of Anglo-Indians, as the half-castes were then called, was now so large that there were fears of an uprising. But they always remained loyal to the British, although they were despised by both British and Indians (Hindu and Muslim). The British barred them from the civil service and most military ranks. But in any emergency they would be mobilized immediately, and relied upon to fight loyally; as soon as the war was over they would be dismissed. With their knowledge of local languages they were employed in businesses all over the country where they were better adapted to the climate than Europeans. From the middle of the nineteenth century they worked particularly on the railways.

Troops were supplied officially for service with local rulers, and their medical officers went with them. The duties were relatively light and these very lucrative posts were hotly competed for. Sometimes the surgeon was asked by a ruler to treat him or his family. The Nizam of Hyderabad was over 80 and very feeble, and, like many of the higher classes of Muslim, he took very large doses of 'provocatives'. He had a paralytic stroke when 'heated'. Indian physicians tried their medicines but without effect. The British surgeon was called. The Nizam recovered and returned to 'his usual indulgences'. After successful treatment, the surgeon might be asked to stay on, and the President would usually raise no objection. The Medical Board might refuse its permission if it would leave them short of staff at the Presidency. The posts were strictly regulated. Head Surgeon Gahagan was sent back to England immediately for visiting His Highness the Nawab of the Carnatic without permission.

Travel through the Company's territory could now be done in comparative safety. But there was still danger in other areas, where:

> a spirit of opposition pervades a large portion of the native population, who are often too adverse to contribute to the comfort, or more properly, to the existence of Europeans.

... It must seem curious that our countrymen are allowed to reside among a people of such a disposition, so far outnumbering us.

The disparity in numbers had always given the British a sense of insecurity, and now there were fears of a general uprising in which they might be overwhelmed.

Communication between Europe and India was now quicker. Attempts were made to shorten the travelling time by exploring overland routes. In the 1770s the Company had control of the Red Sea. If they sailed straight from Bombay to Suez they could then send couriers on to England and get the answers back in half the time. By sea, the ships – the East Indiamen – were larger (1,200-1,400 tons) with a complement of 130, carrying more passengers, and mostly going on to pick up the tea-trade with China. In 1793 the Company had 81,000 tons of shipping, and employed 7,000 seamen. The quickest voyage to Bombay was three months and eighteen days; more usually it took five months. But some voyages were taking much longer,[5] and scurvy was then still a hazard. Travel round the coast of India was dependent on the monsoon – with the monsoon, Madras could be reached from Calcutta in a week; against it, up to three months.

On board, music and dancing helped to keep the men cheerful. The surgeon had time to continue his medical studies although there were distractions such as music, painting, poetry, chess and cards. He had to be on the lookout for shirkers, for whom 'nauseous but innocent' medicines and 'blisters to certain parts that render idleness irksome' were suitable remedies. With the sailors the main problem was drunkenness from hidden stores of liquor. There were always some willing to sell and some to buy, and they would not divulge the source even if 'flogged till they hung senseless at the gangway'. There was plenty of fresh meat for the first week out. After that it was 'corned' (slightly salted), but there were poultry in coops and sheep on hay on the deck so that there was some fresh meat every day. The water was filthy but could be made drinkable by filtering. The usual drink was beer or porter, with spruce beer (each member of the crew got one to two quarts of this daily), lemon juice, and fresh fruit to be made into punch.

Preparations for 'salting' were now started on entering the tropics. Bleeding had been largely abandoned and replaced by purging night and morning, small quantities of meat, alcohol diluted with water, cold baths and light exercise, particularly dancing. On landing, the soldiers, if they were not needed in action, went straight into 'seasoning barracks' for three months. These camps were above sea-level and well away from marshes and the heat and grog-shops of the town. There they had gentle exercise and gradual exposure to the sun; occasional bleeding was required, with tepid bathing and flannel next to the skin.

The British were gradually being convinced of some of the Indian measures against the heat: staying in a darkened apartment, drinking bland fluids, eating a little fruit, perspiring copiously, and not taking a main meal until the evening. Tatties would keep a room 'as cool as Europe'. But it was then dangerous to go out into the heat, particularly between 10 and 4. If this could not be avoided, the chattah (umbrella carried by a servant) was essential. But there were still some, particularly the newcomers and the soldiers,

> who shorten their days by a mode of life unsuitable to the climate; eating great quantities of beef and pork, which the Indian Legislators had wisely forbidden, and drinking copiously of the strong wines of Portugal in the hottest season. They likewise persist obstinately in wearing European dress, which by its ligatures impedes the free circulation of the blood, and by confining the limbs, renders the heat more intolerable.

Higher caste Indians protected themselves with turban and cummerbund. The European equivalent was a large cotton handkerchief folded up in the hat and kept moist, and a fine shawl round the waist. Cotton was preferred to linen as it conducted more slowly. Wool was the same, and 'musical' ladies covered their pianos with blankets in the hot weather. But the torments of the hot weather, with constant irritation from prickly heat, meant that tempers were short. Nearly all the major mutinies occurred at the height of the hot weather, and suicides were more common.

The newcomer was advised to reduce the quantity of his food. Vegetable food was better than animal; he should only have meat after he was 'seasoned'. Much of the meat that was offered for sale was of very poor quality. The village sheep were skeletons full of worms. The alternative was buffalo-beef, 'which might safely be classed as carrion'. Hindus would never sell an ox if they thought it was for slaughter. Gentlemen and regiments had their own flocks, as well as goats, bullocks and pigs. After slaughter, the meat would putrefy in ten hours in spite of all precautions. The Dutch had introduced potatoes and other vegetables from the Cape, and these had now spread all over Bengal. There was plenty of milk; Europeans always sent clean pitchers to the cow.

Breakfast should be early but light, as the stomach could not cope after a bad night, i.e. bread and butter with tea or coffee, but no meat, fish, eggs, or buttered toast. Eggs might be digestible in England, but in India they were a danger to anyone who was bilious. Tiffin (luncheon) should be at 1 o'clock – light curries (spices and condiments only for the seasoned) with a glass or two of wine and some fruit, although the amount of this should be limited in the first year (mangoes caused boils in the unseasoned). Tiffin should be the main meal,[6] and then tea or coffee at 6-7. The bobachee (cook) could be dirty and careless, never tasting the dishes he was preparing, and straining the soup through dirty cloths. There were often flies and dust in everything; the former could be picked out, but the latter made the food uneatable.

The Indian working classes lived entirely on vegetables. They did not have the strength of Europeans but they worked in conditions that would kill a European. They were often addicted to bang, toddy, arrack, or opium. If they kept a strict diet they seemed exempt from many diseases, but when they became ill they had no stamina. The upper classes of Hindus were 'Falstaffs, human porpoises', taking pride in their obesity as a sign of wealth. This was achieved by ghee and indolence, being woken only to drink another cup of ghee, so that they became as bilious as Europeans, and died as early from 'apoplexy, and other fashionable near-cuts to heaven'.

Water for the house was stored in large earthenware jars, in the charge of the aub-dar (who was also an expert at cooling water with saltpetre). These jars filled up in the rains. When larvae appeared they were strained off and a red-hot mass of iron was plunged in followed by alum. A gentleman going out to dinner would then have a supply of this sent ahead with his aub-dar who would cool it and the wine for the dinner-party. For establishments like barracks and hospitals the water came by bullocks carrying two bags of twenty gallons each; these were filled by driving the animals into a pond and baling the water in. For individuals and households the bhisti came with his goatskin bag.[7] He was always a Muslim, as Hindus would not touch animal skins although they might drink from the bag without it touching their lips. In summer he was kept hard at work not only supplying water but watering the tatties from dawn to midnight or longer, sprinkling the floors and surrounds to keep down the dust and accompanying the palanquin on a journey to keep its tatties watered.

Away from home there were even greater hazards from the water. The main source of supply was the 'tank' (artificial pond or lake), often very large, but full of corpses and sometimes alligators; it was used by the locals as a privy, and they would then immerse and wash in it. In the hills the tanks were worse; this was thought to be the reason that the hill men were stunted, with wens, scurvy and ophthalmia. The rivers were no better – as well as partially burnt corpses they might also contain high quantities of chemicals such as copper. No European would drink water that had been freshly drawn in any situation. It always had to stand for at least a day, and then up to one quarter of it might be deposit; it was then boiled.

On campaign, Surgeon Forbes wrote:

> when there is but little water in a leather cantine, the hot wind soon dries it up, and on reaching camp the tank was soon full of elephants, camels, horses, bullocks, men, women and children ... from which with difficulty we strained off a most unpleasant beverage.

Ice had always been available, either made locally by evaporation (p. 65) or by cutting and storing blocks from the hills. Every station had its ice house (deep straw-lined pits).[8]

By the end of the eighteenth century there was a general decrease in heavy drinking among the civilian upper classes in India. Madeira, claret, cider and perry were preferred to spirits, with cooled water at meals, especially with curry. If the object was to keep cool, it was recognized that it was better to avoid stimulating drink. Part of the credit for this was attributed to the captains of the East Indiamen, who inculcated the discipline on the voyage out:

> Rarely indeed does the decanter make more than half a dozen tours (often not so many) after the cloth is removed at dinner, before the company disperses ... after a very frugal supper, the bottle makes a tour or two, when the significant toast of 'Good night, ladies and gentlemen!' sends everyone, at an early hour, to repose. Five or six months of this frugal regimen when approaching the tropics is invaluable.

The soldiers were the exception to this moderation. In the Company the writers worked hard and were temperate, but the military cadets had few duties and spent their time visiting each other and drinking; those who occupied themselves survived. The Navy, also, with less opportunity to learn the changing habits on shore continued with excess of food and drink, and 'do themselves much injury before they see the error'. Liquor was very cheap and 'drunkenness was universal among the lower orders'. The hazards of alcohol in the tropics were well-known. The liability to disease was doubled, and not only were the attacks accelerated but the cure was more difficult and there was a specific effect on the liver. The earliest newspapers (from about 1780) carried warnings every June of the dangers of over-indulgence in the hot season.

But it was agreed that the regular use of wine would relieve the 'torpor and want of tone in the system' produced by the heat. Between meals a little shrub[9] and water or Madeira and water would aid digestion and 'supply the wants of perspiration'. For more serious complaints the value of alcohol was still generally recognized. In India, inflammation was never high enough, even in wounds and ulcers, to be harmed by a moderate use of diluted spirits. The particular benefits were described by Andrew Hunter, Head Surgeon at Berrampore: firstly, the great prostration of the sick in the rainy season; secondly, the depression resulting from low fevers and on recovery from venereal complaints and salivations; thirdly, to make it possible to administer bark; and fourthly, that most soldiers had been long addicted to alcohol, and 'when not administered in sufficient quantity they sink under their disorders'. If wine could not be obtained 'the Men should be supplied with good English beer to the amount of a Quart a day'. Sailors in hospital should be allowed to continue their accustomed grog allowance. Port was valuable in convalescence from bowel complaints. Beer was recommended for scurvy but it was more expensive than wine. Spirits might have to be kept for external application.

Surgeons had to answer charges of over-prescribing and spending too much on bazar medicines and wines, but extra accounts for wine were always passed when it was needed for the sick. The surgeon of the 19th Dragoons, having more sick than usual, ran out of Madeira and used his own stock. His request for a further supply was immediately approved, as the authorities 'did never intend to deprive you of the means of affording every relief to the Sick'. The surgeon justified his actions: 'I will not let lives be lost that otherwise might be saved by the proper Supplies being given me.'

It was laid down that the only wine to be used in the General Hospitals was Madeira at the rate of six dozen per month for twenty men, but only for those 'for whose cure the Surgeon deems it necessary'. The small Regimental Hospitals were not to have any allowance for wine; if the patient had a disorder that needed wine he should be in the General Hospital. On campaign the allowance for the Field Hospitals (Third Mysore War 1790-92) was the same amount of Madeira as at the General Hospitals, with the addition of one dozen of brandy for external use only. Wine was also authorized for the ships carrying recruits, at the rate of one Chest of Port wine for every 80 recruits for use in illness only; any surplus was to be retained for use in the hospitals.

Conditions might remain relatively healthy from the end of July when the plains were flooded, but the expected fevers set in with the November sun when 'evaporation combined with chemicals in the water perform wonders in the cause of desolation'. One of the suggestions for a possible cause of fevers that came to prominence at this time was the 'sol-lunar influence'. Surgeons and their patients had often noticed that fevers reached a peak at the 'full or change' of the moon, or possibly both, with remissions in the inter-lunar periods, and that this might continue for years. Surgeon Francis Balfour, after twenty years in India, described this 'influence' in 1784. He was one of the first to study the fevers of India, and he put forward the thesis, after extensive trials, that the revolutions of the sun and the moon influence disease, accounting for the varieties of fever and the varying severity of smallpox. The human frame was affected by the relative positions of the sun and moon. In health this relation was not strong enough to have obvious effects, but in debility and disease it would 'excite febrile paroxysms'. The moon had a direct influence on fevers and the critical stage was reached when the moon was full or new. The paroxysms might occur every twelve hours, thus also coinciding with the regulation of the tides. He did not claim to know where or how the influence worked. Some surgeons were scornful of his ideas but there were many other people, medical and lay, who were convinced by the regularity of the attacks, and did not necessarily know of Balfour's work. Other trials were carried out on the timing of fevers; some of them showed coincidence. This work attracted much attention which continued into the first quarter of the nineteenth century.

In Britain there was now a greater emphasis on sanitary and public health measures. The old quarantine regulations to prevent the spread of infection were being replaced by sanitary reform, with improved drainage and better housing. This was reflected in the generally diminishing mortality towards the end of the eighteenth century. In India the surgeons repeatedly stressed the dangers of economizing on health measures. It cost far less

> to preserve the life of a Soldier in India, than to supply his place by another from Europe. Even supposing him to be of a constitution so sickly and delicate, as to be obliged to pass a great part of his time in Hospital, many years must elapse, before the expence incurred in this way, will amount to one third the Sum that was required to land him on the Beach of Madras.[10]

The Directors were now asking for more information about conditions in India which might improve medical practice, and the surgeons supplied monthly reports of the morbidity and mortality in hospitals and regiments. In an epidemic all details, dissections (post-mortems), causes and successful treatments were recorded and circulated 'as a guide to future Practitioners'. When it was impossible to control an epidemic among Indian troops, they were sent away from the area on Medical Certificate; this meant that they returned to their homes. If large numbers were sent away, the depleted numbers who remained were overworked. Once at home, many of them rapidly improved. But for those too poor to have any other means of support when they were away from the regiment there were as many deaths as cures.

Conditions in the cities were still noisome. But individual privies were cleaned as soon as they were soiled; there was grass below the seat which was of masonry (wood was too dirty and harboured scorpions). In Calcutta there were continuing complaints about the large burial ground near the centre of the city where the Portuguese buried four hundred bodies a year in shallow graves without coffins. In wet weather some of these appeared above ground and the smell was pestilential. Matter flowing from this got into the tanks:

> laying by this means the foundation of various diseases among the poorer sort of people, who are obliged to drink it; nor can those in more affluent circumstances, from the natural indolence and deception of servants, promise themselves absolute exemption from it.[11]

The Hindus modified their funeral customs for people who died of cholera, smallpox and other contagious diseases, by burying them rather than cremating them, in the belief that

> the ashes of the deceased might be wafted by the winds to other places, and the fell disease spread in all directions.

British ships in harbour had to clear their cables of dead bodies daily.

Even when the health hazards were recognized, there was still the feeling that Indian institutions should be left alone. The care of the individual's body and cleanliness might be laid down by the 'lawgivers of the east', but there were no rules for the lay-out of towns and villages which were usually poorly ventilated, with narrow streets and crowded houses. Nevertheless the magistrates would not interfere with these traditional arrangements. There were no hospitals for Indians, and very few competent Indian medical practitioners.

> The European community ... throughout the country know little, and in fact, have few opportunities of knowing the extent of physical suffering, among the native population in the interior.

But local quarantine precautions were enforced. When a ship arrived with suspected infectious disease on board, a surgeon was sent out to decide whether the crew and passengers were fit to come into the Garrison or whether they should remain in the ship or some other place on shore. There were similar precautions with troops returning from overseas. All clothing was washed, and blankets burned if necessary. But the selected quarantine areas themselves were often notoriously unhealthy, and the medical officers tried to get the troops moved out as soon as possible. Those who remained on the ships in harbour

> are often compelled to take a portion of lascars on board, for the purpose of aiding those who survive the pestilental miasma, to which they are so inconsiderately, or, more properly, inhumanly subjected ... those who escape with their lives, are usually much weakened by severe attacks of the ague.

There were no separate hospitals for civilians. The General Hospitals took all European patients, civil, military and naval, and also European paupers. All who could afford it were charged for attendance and accommodation. The soldiers might be reluctant to come into hospital unless they were seriously ill as it meant giving up their accustomed liquor. But they also tended to use the hospital to escape their duties. The surgeons were warned to be on the look-out for abuse of the system, and to ensure that the old lags were not admitted, 'where they acquire sluggish and indolent habits extremely detrimental to Military Discipline'.

Some of the hospitals were in poor repair and there were complaints from the surgeons:

> It is universally allowed that Sobriety, fresh air and cleanness are of as much, or perhaps more consequence in the prevention and cure of deseases than either Diet or Medicines.

In Calcutta the wards could not be kept dry and clean, and the atmosphere was contaminated by 'the Stench of the necessaries fitted up under the same roof'. The boundary wall was so imperfect that no sentry could prevent access to the 'numerous arrack shops with which the hospital is surrounded' so that the soldiers could get liquor 'whenever they think proper'.

The equipment needed for each sick man in hospital, his clothes, bedding, and victuals, were all carefully specified. Mattresses were abandoned as dirty and harbouring infection. Hospital clothing was made of gingham, and the cots were taped (instead of rattan), so that mattresses were not needed and everything could be washed. There was one attendant for every six men, and one for any single man when the surgeon thought it necessary. There were assistants to help prepare the medicines. The wards were fumigated with benjamin [benzoin] and sprinkled with vinegar twice a week from April to November and once a week the rest of the year.

The diets were now standardized throughout the three Presidencies as full, middle, milk, and low. On a full diet breakfast and supper consisted of rice made into congee with milk. Dinner was one pound of bread (if not available, boiled rice) and usually mutton (regarded as the best form of meat for Europeans in a hot climate): 'one joint of Mutton at the rate of one Sheep to every eight men' with soup which should contain 'Greens Onions and Black pepper'. On the middle diet the mutton was reduced to half a joint. The milk diet consisted of rice and milk only, with one pound of bread. On the low diet there was 12 oz. bread or rice with salt fish for dinner, but otherwise as the full diet. Debilitated patients were given one pint of tea, 'limon grass tea' or sago for breakfast and supper with one chicken or chicken broth and sago or pudding for dinner and 12 oz. bread a day. For every patient, whatever the diet, there was a daily allowance of salt and sugar with 'congee water' made from boiled rice as the common drink and a supply of 'good' water. Sometimes the diets included two spoonfuls of Madeira. Wine and spirits were added as prescribed by the surgeon.

The prevailing diseases in 284 patients at the Military Hospital in Madras, for one month in 1782, were: venereals 50, fevers 37, simple fluxes 20, fluxes complicated with liver and visceral obstruction 177. In the same period the Naval Hospital had twice the number of patients, many of whom had been admitted with ulcers of the legs (p. 140), but very few venereals. The sailors had little communication with the shore and no prize money, and 'the easy ladies at Madras do not often venture on the ships'.

Clinical trials of drugs, either sent out from England or collected locally, were carried out at the General Hospitals. The advantage of using soldiers for these trials was that they could be followed up by the regimental surgeons after discharge from hospital. Samples of all products likely to be useful were sent out to Head Surgeons for their comments and further trials. A styptic solution arrived with a favourable report from England but the surgeons found that it was no better than dry lint for stopping external bleeding and that it was useless internally for spitting blood. A new species of bark sent in by William Roxburgh (p. 240) with the suggestion that it might be a 'substitute for the Peruvian' was found to be effective. A remedy for snake-bite from Tanjore was supported by C. F. Swartz, a well-known missionary, who had often seen it administered successfully, but it was found to contain high levels of arsenic. James Anderson, the Physician General, put in a strongly critical minute:

> Two thirds of our snakes are not venomous and if these pills are administered to all that are bit, three persons must run the risque of their lives, under the Idea of saving one by a Dose of Arsenic.

But Head Surgeon Duffin had given it to more than fifty patients without ill effects. He accepted that the pills contained arsenic, but there was no means of knowing enough about the vegetable substances with which it was compounded to know whether they would modify the toxic action. He thought that each practitioner should be left to use his own discretion.

A frequent cause of admission to hospital was punishment by flogging. The 'punished men' gave the surgeons not only a great deal of extra work but extra expense for the bulky dressings needed for the huge open wounds. There were frequent complaints from the surgeons that the daily allowance that they received for each sick man was not enough to cover this. Indians were flogged with rattans which splintered, causing irritation and death from 'a locked jaw' (tetanus). These complications were due to the method and not to the severity of the punishment in which up to 40 stripes were inflicted. The full punishment in the British Army, carried out by the regimental drummers, was 1,000 lashes, and some men could stand this without dying. When the Royal troops arrived in India in the middle of the eighteenth century they were known as 'bloody-backs' from the frequency of official floggings. The victims were 'forced to keep their beds for several weeks, and most like to Die; Neither could any of 'em ease Nature, or make Water, for several days.' Discipline was always less severe in the Company's armies. Flogging was abolished for sepoys in 1827, except for stealing, marauding, or gross insubordination. The cat-of-nine-tails was substituted for the rattan which was abolished in 1828 as 'occasioning serious bodily injury, far beyond the intention of the law'. Flogging was abolished in the Indian Army by Bentinck in 1835, but continued in the British Army, although the number of lashes was limited.

Ulcers of the legs were a common cause of disability. Many of them were venereal or due to chronic wound infections and osteomyelitis; some were tuberculous or varicose. There were also a large number occurring at sea in young sailors. At the Naval Hospital in Madras in 1782 'the great bulk of cases consisted at all times of ulcers'. As the north-east monsoon set in in October all amputation stumps, sores and ulcers got worse, but all improved with the cooler, drier weather of December. There was often 'a latent scorbutic taint'. Fresh meat and vegetables were scarce at the time from the plundering of the surrounding country by Haider Ali's troops (p.127). The connection between scurvy and leg ulcers was clear to all naval surgeons, and the incidence of these ulcers decreased as scurvy was brought under control.

There were frequent reports of outbreaks of 'malignant ulcer' (hospital gangrene) with large foul ulcers arising from the slightest injury, and rapidly going on to gangrene. This was spread by careless attendants with dirty sponges and bandages, and the stench in the ward would become unsupportable. All dressings were to be destroyed and never used a second time, even after washing. The incidence of gangrene was closely related to diet, and in an epidemic, improvement would follow a change to a more nutritious diet. It was a common complication of ulceration of the legs, as in Indian prisoners chafed by their fetters; many of them were undernourished, probably suffering from sub-clinical scurvy. There were many more ulcers among the sepoys than in the convicts in hospital. The sepoys would refuse food that might cure their ulcers but was against their caste-rules. The lower-caste convicts had no such scruples. In war-wounds hospital gangrene was common; it was very painful and carried a high mortality. Only a few were saved by amputation, but even if they died their last hours had been made easier by changing their agonizing pain to 'the more endurable suffering of a simple incised wound'.

Formerly it was thought that a 'simple' [varicose] ulcer acted as an outlet for 'acrid humours in the blood'. If the ulcer healed, the disordered humours would cause serious complications. If it looked like healing, the danger could be avoided by opening an 'issue' in some other part of the body – usually a 'pea-issue', formed by incising a fold of skin and inserting a number of peas to keep it open. But as belief in the 'humoral' basis of medicine died out (p. 81) it was regarded as safe to heal ulcers. It was recognized that they would heal if the leg was kept horizontal but that they would always break down again when the patient started to walk, unless the leg was firmly bandaged with adhesive strips. The influence of varicose veins was controversial, and surgeons tried the effect of various methods of ligaturing the veins in the leg. But there were many complications, and operative treatment was condemned.[12]

When a war was expected, detailed instructions were issued for setting up Field Hospitals. The transport required for the sick and wounded for an army of 10,000, of which 4,000 were Europeans, was 320 doolies[13] with 1,600 bearers, 120 wagons with 400 bullocks, 5 superintendents for the doolies, and 5 for the wagons, a smith and a carpenter, each with 10 men, with additional rattan men (to make splints) and tailors, 12 tents for the sick, and two marquees for preparing medicines, and for the attendants to sleep in. When the army halted the poles were taken out of the doolies so that they could be used as cots. Conditions were always worse for the troops in the monsoon. There were often not enough cots, and the surgeons complained that the patients had to sleep on the sodden ground. In general, the sick rate was always lower in the better disciplined regiments which insisted on higher standards of hygiene. This was accentuated by the differing mortality in the infantry and the cavalry on campaign. The infantry sent their sick to hospital and suffered the usual high death rate. The cavalry carried their sick with them and the death rate was lower. After a battle, Surgeon James Forbes wrote:

we remained the next day to perform the necessary amputations, and administer such comfort as we could to the sick and wounded; our flying hospital now consisting of more than four hundred patients, most of them in violent fevers in consequence of the extreme heat and the wounds received.

The continuous military action was causing more complaints at home. The stockholders were getting anxious, and there was a general feeling that all the Company's affairs were corrupt. An Act of 1774 established Parliament's authority to interfere in the Company's administration and to support the rights of Indians. The Company instituted reforms in India but continued to enlarge its territories and political influence. In the first half of the nineteenth century its powers would gradually be taken over by Parliament.

Notes

1 This period has been called 'the Rape of Bengal'.

2 The Company took over the police in 1790 and the jails in 1792. Up to 1793 Indians guilty of dacoity (robbery by armed gangs) were handed over to Muslim courts. Their right hands and left feet were dissected off through the joint (each limb took three minutes); the stumps were dressed with boiling ghee, and the parts were thrown in the river. This was abolished by the British, and imprisonment substituted.

3 The Company did not take over the civil administration of Bengal until 1772.

4 An independent trader with a grudge against the Company.

5 Clive's first voyage out had taken from 10 March 1743 to 1 June 1744.

6 An alternative menu for a lunch party from about the same time consisted of soup, roast fowl, curry and rice, a mutton pie, a fore-quarter of lamb, a rice pudding, tarts, very good cheese, and excellent Madeira.

7 *bhishti*, 'a person of paradise' (Pers). His bag was the whole skin of a large goat. Gunga Din was a regimental bhisti (Kipling).

8 From 1833 cargoes of ice from America were shipped to Calcutta.

9 Fruit juice and spirit.

10 Each soldier had cost the Company £100 by the time he reached his Corps in India.

11 The first house tax for repairing and cleaning the streets was introduced in 1794. No major improvements were made until 1835.

12 The true pathology of the veins of the leg was not worked out until the twentieth century.

13. *doli*, a covered litter (Hind.). One report (in England) of a battle in India stated that 'ferocious Doolies rushed down from the hills and carried off the wounded'.

IV
ORIENTALISM 1780-1835

Chapter Ten
Reforms in India

In 1773 the Company had to borrow money from Parliament. Lord North offered a large loan but insisted on a Bill to change the constitution of the Company. As part of this Regulating Act, which came into force in 1774, Warren Hastings was appointed Governor-General. From his earlier time in India (from 1758) Hastings had continually protested at the plundering of Bengal. On his arrival for the second time there were military and financial crises. His task was made worse by the disastrous famine of 1770 (p. 127). But by the time he left (1785) Bengal was more prosperous than it had ever been. Clive had won power for the Company, but Hastings, who was the last of the Company's servants to be wholly trained in its service, started the reforms that would turn the traders into civil servants.

Pitt's India Bill (1784) set up a Board of Control, with members appointed by the Crown, to control the political, military and revenue sides of the Company's activities, but not to interfere in commercial affairs. The tea-voyages to China were now the Company's most profitable trade. In 1767 Parliament had imposed duties on various imports into the American colonies, which were all repealed in 1770 except the duty on tea in the interests of the Company. By the Tea Act (1773) tea was to be sent straight from India to America so that the Americans had to pay tax.[1]

Cornwallis was sent out to India in 1785 to continue the reforms, bringing with him independent officials and judges of the High Court. The administration was taken into British hands, and independent courts of justice were set up. Company servants who had been heavily involved in private trading were sent home. British officials were installed at the head of every department, and all Indian officials were strictly supervised.[2]

There were new regulations for the medical services. Hospital and Medical Boards were set up in each of the three Presidencies to be responsible for all the Company's medical services in the area. The Boards' instructions from the Directors were, firstly, to reduce expenses, and then to ensure that the sick and wounded were properly attended to, and 'gross abuses chequed of receiving into the Hospitals men with trivial complaints'. There were new conditions of employment. Up to then the surgeons had been employed on 'warrant', thus ranking as warrant officers below the most junior army subalterns. In 1788 the warrants were withdrawn and they were awarded Commissions, starting with the pay and emoluments of captains.

Medical officers could choose whether to belong to the civil or the military branches. Cornwallis emphasized the obligation to serve and not to stay in 'civil stations of ease and emolument'.[3] Military duties always had priority, and all surgeons were ordered to have a period of military duty before any civilian appointment. The newly-arrived surgeon had to complete eighteen months as a Hospital Mate (Assistant Surgeon) before he was eligible for any other duty, and usually he would be required to spend a further two to three years on military service before being offered any civilian post. Private trading was abolished, but salaries were raised to bring them into line with their army equivalents. Regimental Surgeons were allowed a fixed sum for each sick man treated in barracks. Stoppages from each sepoy's pay were made to cover the Indian doctor of each battalion and the supply of 'country and bazar' medicines, so that no further allowance for these was given. But the Assistant Surgeon should 'afford them whatever Europe Medicines he may think necessary'.

Before this there were no pensions and no home leave. Now, long service became the rule with three years home leave after ten years service. Military and medical personnel were allowed pensions, but civil servants had large salaries and fees, and were expected to return home with 'competent fortunes'. Funds were set up for invalids, widows and orphans. The earliest was Lord Clive's Fund (1770) when Clive handed over to the Company the five lakhs (c. £63,000) in money and jewels bequeathed to him by Mir Jafar, the Nawab of Moorshedabad. From this a Colonel received £228, a Captain and a Surgeon £91, a Lieutenant and an Assistant Surgeon £45 per annum, and a Private 6*d.* per day (9*d.* if he had lost a limb). Later, there were subscription Funds (1804) and Funds to which all officers were required to contribute (1820). Pensions for soldiers' wives only continued for six months, and the children's allowance stopped at fourteen. The boys could either enlist or become apprenticed as compounders and dressers in the Subordinate Medical Department, and the girls were expected to marry early or they would starve or turn to prostitution.

Soldiers who were not fit for full duty were placed in the Invalid Corps where they carried out light duties. This Corps catered for 'the debauched as well as the honorably wounded' so that alcoholics were included. This did not apply to civilians – the drunks were cut out of polite society and quickly finished up in their graves. Soldiers who were unfit for all duties were classified as Pensioners. They needed more medical care than the Invalids, 'many of them without legs and arms, with stiff joints and variously maimed'. These pension arrangements also applied to the sepoys and their Indian doctors. Many of the latter had served long and faithfully, and they were always supported in their pension claims by the surgeons under whom they had worked.

In 1778 a scheme was started to give members of the Invalid Corps of sepoys plots of land to go back to husbandry with their families. The plots were so sited that the old soldiers could form a line of protection against marauding mountain tribes. This scheme worked successfully, but gradually died out after 1821 by which time the warlike hill-people 'by kind and humane treatment after they had been controlled' had been induced to come down and settle in the villages.

Up to now, European interest in India had been primarily commercial, although intelligent travellers had recognized the antiquity of Indian culture. Captain Niebuhr, in Bombay in 1763 as an envoy of the King of Denmark, reported:

> the Indians are, besides, the most ancient of the nations whose history is known ... examination further would be worthy of a prince or a whole nation; the Portuguese and the British have done nothing.

Now the philosophical 'Enlightenment' in Europe was bringing about social and political changes which, from the 1780s, began to have their effects in India. The new liberalism and humanitarianism brought increasing interest in Indian history and culture, including medicine.

Warren Hastings had been the first to encourage these subjects by founding the Madrassa (Muslim College) in Calcutta in 1781 at his own expense for the study of languages and law by Indians. The Sanskrit College of Benares was set up in 1791 by Jonathan Duncan,[4] the Resident at Benares, with support from Cornwallis, to study science and medicine. The teaching was largely by Company officers, partly in English and partly in the vernaculars. Scholars in the Company – notably Sir William Jones and Sir Charles Wilkins – translated Sanskrit works of astronomy, mathematics, medicine and literature. These translations began to appear in 1789, and Europeans were astonished to learn of the antiquity of Indian culture, science and medicine.

Knowledge of India was increased when the Company gave permission to a number of British artists to travel widely in India, producing not just portraits of prominent individuals but scenes of different parts of India – the 'Indian Picturesque'. There was a general revival of interest in Indian Medicine. Classical Ayurveda was recognized as similar to the brunonian system which played an important part in the medical thinking of the eighteenth century in England (p. 109)

The most important figure in this 'orientalist' movement was Sir William Jones who had started the study of oriental languages at school. From 1775-83 he was a barrister in London. During this time he published translations of Persian, Turkish and Arabic literature. In 1783 he went to India as puisne [junior] Judge in Bengal. On the voyage he conceived the idea of an Asiatic Society to study all aspects of Indian culture. The Asiatick Society was founded in 1784 with him as its first President. He found that the legal system for Hindus was based on a traditional text which was interpreted erratically by the brahmins. To regularize this he started to learn Sanskrit. The problem was to get access to the necessary books; it was sacrilege for the brahmins to let a foreigner even see them. Gradually he won their confidence, and they co-operated with him to produce a legal code which was published by the Government in Calcutta in 1794.

Jones encouraged the study of Indian Medicine and its drugs and herbs. He founded *Asiatick Researches* in 1789 to make all new information more widely known. 'Discourse the Eleventh', which he gave before the Society in February 1794, contained his thoughts on the value of Indian Medicine. He also contributed papers on elephantiasis[5] and snake-bite. He argued that there was much to be gained from a study of the plants of India for their medicinal as well as their commercial value. He set out in detail how this should be done in 'The Design of a Treatise on the Plants of India', although he deplored the use of sexual metaphors by the classical botanists, as 'inflaming the imagination and unfit for women' — some of the descriptions could not be read in English. At the same time he was translating the classics of Sanskrit literature. These were not only widely acclaimed in Europe but made available to Indians knowledge of their own culture which had been kept secret by the brahmins. Translations of his work into other European languages, particularly German, stimulated studies of Indology in European universities. Jones died of hepatitis on 27 April 1794 and was buried in Calcutta. He had always urged greater understanding of Indians, but his original proposal to admit Indians to the Asiatick Society was not adopted until 1820. The first paper by an Indian was read in 1784 but the author was not admitted.

Jones and his supporters felt that Indian culture should not be interfered with, but that as much as possible should be learned from it. Indian institutions should, as far as possible, be left alone (the preoccupation with Hindu culture at this time tended to neglect the Muslim). This policy was applied even when there were health hazards, as in poorly ventilated and crowded streets and houses where the thatched roofs caused many fires. Some of the houses were so damp that seeds swept into a corner would germinate. Attempts to introduce improvements were often frustrated by adherence to old customs. But when some streets in Calcutta were widened in 1790 the initial outcry changed when it was seen how health and convenience had improved. For the customs of suttee (p. 45) and infanticide (p. 218) the British tried to reason with Hindu leaders to persuade them that these were later additions and not part of pure Hindu tradition. This had some success around Bombay, but, in the 1820s, more than 6,000 cases of suttee were recorded around Calcutta. Governor Bentinck's Act making suttee illegal was introduced in 1829 without major disturbance.

When the Company took over the jails in 1792 conditions were appalling, with large numbers of prisoners and a high mortality. The general standard of health was low. The prisoner was separated from his family who would probably starve in his absence. He himself, if not indigent before, had become so from the wholesale bribery required throughout his trial. He had been moved out of his familiar surroundings – the effect of this was most noticeable in men from the hills. Many were addicted to opium, other drugs and tobacco, and the deprivation of these added to their miseries. In the unhealthy climate of the jail they were more liable to any infectious disease. They were exhausted after a day of hard manual labour wearing chains weighing seven pounds or more. Two-thirds of the admissions to hospital were due to chafing from the leg irons, and this often led to hospital gangrene (p. 140). It was noted that debtors, lunatics and women, who were not sentenced to hard labour, did much better than the men. Before it was abolished, the effects of corporal punishment had also been a frequent cause of admission to hospital (p. 140). But now the care of prisoners came to be part of the duties of the civil medical officers who were required to furnish regular reports. An Indian doctor was appointed to accompany any gang of prisoners who were detached for any length of time beyond the reach of immediate assistance from the medical officer.

The British were beginning to take some responsibilty for the people they were governing. The officials, a new class of very able adminstrators, tried to govern in harmony with Indian feelings, only introducing improvements that the Indians would accept, and slowly preparing them for self-government. Sir Thomas Munro, the popular Governor of Madras, foresaw that 'the time would come when England would withdraw from India'. He advised the Company that:

> your rule is alien and it can never be popular ... you are not here to turn India into England or Scotland. Work through, not in spite of, native systems and native ways, with a prejudice in their favour rather than against them; and when ... your subjects can frame and maintain a worthy Government for themselves, get out and take ... the sense of having done your duty as the chief reward for your exertions.

Lord Wellesley (Governor-General 1798) had proposed a training college for all civil servants on arrival in India to study the vernaculars and Indian law and literature. Because this was ruled by the Directors as too expensive it was restricted to Bengal where Fort William College was opened in 1800 with a staff that included Indian scholars. Young Indians gradually became involved and the liberal ideas that they learned there were to lead to the rise of nationalism and the demand for Home Rule (p.227). In 1828 the College was abolished and the new administrators were sent at once to their stations where moonshees[6] were provided for teaching the local languages. They now had regular higher salaries and increasing authority over enormous areas; they had to learn that each area had its own customs and that policy had to be adapted to suit. They were in close contact with the local rulers and zemindars,[7] and it was essential for them to be fluent in the local language.

At home the Company founded Haileybury College in 1805 to educate its future civil servants. The education at home and the subsequent training in India led to the development of strong family links and traditions with the emphasis on service to India and its people.[8]

The first official move by the Company to educate Indians came in the Charter of 1813 with the grant of one lakh[9] of rupees; all previous efforts had been made by individual Company officers. Colleges were set up, mainly in Bengal with the help of wealthy Indians; the emphasis was on English. At first there were strong prejudices among Indians against English education but this changed when it was seen that it would lead to employment by the Government. Bengal was the first to develop a new middle class of minor officials. Muslims were slower to take advantage of this new policy, and Hindus thus gained an increased status.

The British recognized that there had been a strong tradition of science in India in the past. Astronomy had been one of the main areas. In the early eighteenth century Maharajah Jai Singh II of Jaipur had built five observation posts in different parts of India using huge instruments of masonry of perfect stability. But, in general, the British thought that Indian science was in decline and they regarded their own as far superior. They admired the skills of Indian craftsmen, but they found them lacking in originality and creativity, simply following the customs of their ancestors and being expert at exact copying. So they were surprised to find that the quality of steel and fabrics produced in India was superior to theirs, and that Indian dyeing techniques were far ahead of the European. There were problems of learning these techniques from Indians who were naturally secretive. Attempts to set up new industries in India were limited by the fear that they would interfere with trade at home. From 1780 excellent ships were being built in India, but after 1830 the Company stopped this in order to keep full employment of shipwrights at home. Although in the past, surgical instruments had been expertly made, the British were still sending their old instruments back to England for repair; the Company had its own cutler in London. Instruments rusted rapidly in India but they 'would have been serviceable if there had been a Cutler established here'.

From 1760 there had been a rapid increase in the number of Europeans in India. By the beginning of the nineteenth century the population of Calcutta was 100,000, of whom 1,000 were British.

The Company's regulations were published yearly from 1810 in the *East India Directory*, and everyone was expected to obey them, including the ban on horse-racing on Sunday, but church-going was now 'unfashionable'. Some of the highest officials, notably Cornwallis, lived austere and overworked lives, but below them there was a flourishing social life. There were elaborate dinners and balls. Ladies who danced through the night were in danger of 'consumptions' by going out on to the verandah. There were theatres for professionals and amateurs, and regimental stations ran their own theatricals. In the coffee-houses one rupee would bring a dish of coffee and the newspapers, English as well as Indian. There were racecourses and a wide range of sporting activities, from tiger shooting to mountain climbing, and these were another cause of fatalities. The English in India

> pursued their sports with a desperate disregard for the customs of the country ... the climate had taught Indians for countless generations that passivity was the answer.

Some of the officers owned yachts, and there were boating parties. Cricket was not popular; the alternate exertion and inactivity gave rise to severe colds which could lead to serious illness.

'The absence of elderly persons in Indian society, is one of the first things that strike a new arrival.' But young unmarried women were also very scarce. By 1810 there were still only 250 European women in Bengal, while there were 4,000 respectable men, civilian and military, many of whom could not afford to get married, with the number of servants, carriages etc. that were expected. It was the custom for the men, at all social levels, to keep an Indian woman. A concubine was preferable to marriage to an Indian which was strongly discouraged by the Government. A woman 'under the protection of an English gentleman' was regarded as though she was married to him, but, however highly born, she was never invited to official functions. The expenses of concubinage were calculated at Rs. 40/month (£60/year), and this information was included in official publications with a note that, although this might seem a heavy charge, it was cheap compared with supporting a British lady. Below the rank of major, permission for an officer to marry was required from the Governor. Private soldiers were allowed to marry, but most of them had a companion. There were very few European women with the regiments, and Indian women gave invaluable help when their men were ill. The number of British women in India rapidly increased through the early part of the nineteenth century. The possibilities of an early advantageous marriage led to large numbers of young women going out to India to take their chance. On reaching India they could expect 'three hundred a year, dead or alive' – on marriage a civil servant was guaranteed at least £300 a year and his widow would get a similar pension when he died.

Children were expensive. They all had to be sent home – few stayed in India after they were three or four years old. This cost £100 and the same or more for an attendant. They should have had smallpox (or vaccination), measles and whooping cough before the voyage, in case they might in England 'be carried off by them, thus rendering all their parents' anxiety, and possibly their ill-spared disbursements, of no avail'. The mother's ill-health might mean that she had to go too, so that the family would be broken up until the husband could save enough to go home. It was now Company policy that all its military personnel should subscribe to the Orphan Fund that had been started in 1782. Orphaned girls were poorly provided for, but the sons of officers were apprenticed to business, and the sons of soldiers to the regiments as drummers and fifers.

In the hot weather moderate perspiration was always thought to be beneficial. There was a 'sympathy' between the secretions of the skin and the stomach which promoted good health. The newcomer changed his shirt three or four times a day but this only made the perspiration worse. A shirt carefully dried and worn again once or twice was acceptable and caused less perspiration than a fresh one. The obligatory morning ride was taken in the previous evening's linen and not changed until after breakfast. Ladies' stays were made so that the servant could move the bones from one pair to another in a few minutes, and ladies could change their stays when they changed their linen.

It was the rule to wear uniform on all public occasions, and 'for gentlemen to meet in society without cloth coats would be highly improper'; there was the risk that Europeans might not be respected in any other dress. For the soldiers it was a matter of pride to make no concessions to the heat, and they 'existed in a kind of warm bath (unpleasant for them and their neighbours)'. In 1813 there was a general order that any officer on leave not in proper uniform would be sent back to his regiment. As late as 1827 all officers were ordered to wear regulation dress (of official broadcloth) in public. Indian soldiers were equally determined to keep their tight-fitting uniforms. This meant that they could not sit down without unbuttoning their pantaloons, and to pick something off the ground they had pass it to their hands with their feet.

But customs were changing, and evening visiting was now more relaxed so that coats were dispensed with, and only an upper and an under waistcoat of white linen were worn, the former having sleeves. The new arrivals, at first 'sticklers for decorum', soon fell in with this and took off their coats after the first civilities, putting on a waistcoat that a servant had ready for them.

With the general decrease in alcohol consumption, tippling between meals – earlier recommended (p. 134) – was now not respectable. It continued in the punch-houses, but 'no European of character would be seen there, and the habit would exclude him from all social intercourse'. Newcomers were advised to bring letters of introduction with them so that they could be invited at once into a gentleman's house and so avoid the perils of the punch-house. But cheap liquor was available in large quantities. Ten million gallons of spirits were made or sold in Bengal in a year; there were abundant licences for the retail of spirits and 'an incalculable number of shops'. There were 600 liquor shops in Madras, many of them near the hospital. This was in addition to the amount imported and sold each year in Calcutta: four thousand pipes each of madeira and claret, and ten thousand gallons of brandy, hollands, and rum.

The continuing high incidence of disease in the troops was ascribed to alcohol. The Surgeon General's Report for 1802 stated:

> the prevailing diseases of His Majesty's Scotch Brigade are attributed to the immoderate use of Arrack and exposure afterwards to the Night Air. Most of the diseases of His Majesty's 74th regiment are likewise considered.

The private soldiers, living with Indian women, often in squalid conditions, were always more liable to disease than their officers with their better diet and housing. The problems of troops retained for too long in particularly unhealthy areas were now recognized, and it became the policy to move them at regular intervals. In October 1787 Cornwallis ordered a General Relief of the Troops at the several Stations of the Army. Notice was given that a similar relief would take place every year at about the same time.

The treatment of diseases in their seasonal pattern was now standardized, and would remain almost unchanged for many years.[10]

> India diseases are so simple and vary so little that large numbers can be treated in a way that elsewhere would be incompatible with due attention and care.

The simple precautions necessary to avoid disease, or at least to mitigate the effects, were given in medical texts, and now also in the writings of experienced non-medical travellers. But death could occur suddenly, at all ages, with a fit like apoplexy that had 'no deference to the abstemious and temperate, any more than to the licentious and gourmandizing classes'. Constitution seeemed to have little to do with it; the strongest were often in the most danger. Newcomers suffered for their contempt of what they regarded as 'luxurious and effeminate practices'. They refused to be carried about in palankeens, or to use chattahs, and took their accustomed exercise in the heat of the day. This activity continued until 'some climate sickness is brought on, and teaches them', or even 'made it necessary to attend their funerals'.

It was important to control the amount of perspiration – too little would result in diseases due to the heat, but too much would weaken the system. Women who led an indolent life with little exercise were liable to 'convulsions, spasms, and other hysteric symptoms'. The 'consent of parts' or 'sympathy', although unexplained, was particularly important in the tropics. The sympathy of the stomach with the skin warned that one must not eat too much in the heat, and must rest before dinner. There was also characteristic overactivity of the liver resulting in increased secretion of bile. This cutaneo-hepatic sympathy was one of the strongest in the human frame, so that perspiration was a certain index of biliary flow, and to check the former would moderate the latter. Over-stimulation of the liver would lead to irregular secretion of vitiated bile which caused 'irregularity, languor, nausea, a yellowish complexion, a poor appetite, and a feeling of boiling lead flowing throught the intestines'. These biliary disorders were 'the grand sources of almost every disease that occurs'. Temperance in all things was recognized as the most important measure, and the virtues of the Hindu were again extolled.

The Hindus were seen to be personally clean, living in huts which allowed a free flow of air, rather than the closed stone houses of the Europeans. They slept on mats, not beds, and the stove was movable, so that the whole building was fumigated. The floor and walls were smeared with cow-dung which was thought to be antiseptic. Outside the huts, vultures, butcher-birds, pariah dogs and jackals acted as scavengers. The lower castes smoked constantly, and the tobacco was thought to help their resistance to disease. They ate no meat so that there were no shambles as a source of putrefaction. There were no privies, but they all went outside the city for their morning ritual. In the four months after the rains there were dangerous vapours in the evenings. In the cities these were countered by the general fumigation of the fires for the evening meal at 6 or 7 o'clock. But the effects were much worse in the villages, with fevers on and off for years, commonly at full or change of the moon. Whole villages could be affected.

They die, almost without any pain, in the same manner as consumptive persons; and become extinct like a lamp which has no longer oil. They never whimper or complain, like so many of the Europeans, who quit the world in the most painful manner imaginable.

The main hazard was the water supply. Most epidemics were believed to be air-borne, especially cholera, and there were few precautions with the water. Maternal mortality was high. The midwives came from the lowest castes (p. 104). Many births were held to be doomed as 'unlucky'. Anyone who had been lucky enough to be born feet first might be called upon to jump seven times over the woman in labour. If there was a wet-nurse, she was chosen with care; all her family were considered as relatives, so that the child could not marry the nurse's children.

Before 1792, when the first hospital for Indian civilians was opened in Calcutta, there was no regular provision for the medical treatment of Indians who were not in the service of the Company. There was continuing debate as to how far medical resources should be stretched to cover Indian civilians. The Government was increasingly urging the surgeons to treat all classes of Indians, but the surgeons were concerned that this might interfere with their primary responsibility to the army. They also knew from experience that it was usually only the poorest Indians who would apply for, and accept, treatment from a European. Both Hindus and Muslims were now more ready to call on British surgeons but there were still taboos in the higher castes.[11] It might be difficult to persuade a brahmin to take Peruvian bark or any medicine if it was mixed with alcohol, but mixed in water or with ingredients familiar to him it was acceptable. Other castes were less particular if they were assured that the prescription would bring about a cure. But they were all strongly opposed to 'post-mortem researches'.

For the hospital, the Town Major would consult with the surgeon to work out the charges, and the patient was then given a certificate of admission. European medicines were available for Indian civilians for payment as outpatients. In August 1786 the Company made a profit of 25 per cent on the sale of medicines from the Company's stores to the inhabitants of Calcutta. Any Indian who was brought in badly injured or diseased was not to be turned away. An immediate certificate could be granted, but the matter should then be reported to Government. The lascars (sailors) from the ships in harbour were also to be admitted, but each patient had to bring a certificate from the Town Major. The medical authorities were always careful to give priority to employees of the Company.

Regimental surgeons in country districts were often overwhelmed with requests for medical help by the local inhabitants. It was official policy to encourage this, both to promote goodwill for the Company's political aims and as part of the growing feeling of responsibility for all Indians in areas under Company rule. The local problems could be exacerbated by the numbers of pilgrims passing through the district, bringing with them new and epidemic diseases (p. 88). One surgeon to an Indian battalion sent in a request for more resources as he had to cope with 30,000 pilgrims a year. Many of them applied to him for medical assistance, and 'their condition was so shocking that he felt that he could not withhold aid'.

It was assumed that the Hindu would withstand surgical operations, and recover from the effects of injury, better than the over-fed alcoholic European soldier. As an example of the rapid healing of wounds in Hindus, the religious exercise of 'hook swinging'[12] was quoted. If the flesh gave way and the man fell, the wound in his back would heal more quickly than expected. Hindus were able to make long journeys carrying heavy loads in the heat, but this was not necessarily due to their abstemious habits. Many of them, being of low caste, would eat and drink anything they could get hold of, and they relied on opium for their stamina (p. 245). Surgeons found that, for a European, they had to 'lower the temperament to repress the tendency to inflammation', whereas, in a Hindu, supportive measures were needed to 'prevent his sinking'. This was even more marked when they started to treat the inhabitants of large cities and in Bengal, where the standard of health of the general population was low. Country-dwellers, sepoys and prisoners in British jails[13] did better, but even in the soldiers it was noticed on some of the campaigns that surgical operations were less successful in Indians than in Europeans. Indian troops, if moved out of their accustomed surroundings, were particularly susceptible to the diseases of the new area. Sepoys moving from the plains into the hills would succumb to Hill Fever. There was also the problem of taking them overseas (p. 121). In observance of their taboos they were allowed to carry their own water and provisions. The water on board was kept in large teak tanks, and the sepoys would take all precautions to prevent it from impure contact. Even so, some of them would not drink it or eat food made with it. The casks were taboo if they had previously contained spirits or meat. On many occasions it was noted that, when provisions did not last through the voyage, the sepoys would go for days 'almost expiring from thirst and want of nourishment'.[14]

The Native Hospital in Calcutta in 1792 was supported by public and private subscriptions. It was staffed by Company surgeons, supplied with medicines from the Company Dispensatory, and managed by equal numbers of European and Indian Governors. The original plan was to build a series of huts, housing 300 patients, and not costing more than £2,000 a year. But a more permanent building was agreed, and the extra expense of this limited the number of patients.[15] In the 1790s public lotteries were held in Calcutta, and churches, the town hall and canals were built with the proceeds. But the Committee of the Native Hospital, with a strong missionary influence, refused this lottery money for their hospital.[16] There was a feeling that the local wealthy Indians could have done more to support the hospital, and that larger donations might have been expected 'from that spontaneous flow of genuine humanity, with which the Hindu code is replete'. It would make a change from them building 'immense houses, richly endowed, for the maintenance of an idle gang of priests'.

Indents for 'medicines and implements' were passed by the Hospital Board. Regular Hindu attendants were appointed, and regular supplies of water from the Ganges made available. For the year 1797 there were 209 in-patients and 464 out-patients; 523 had been discharged, 36 had died, and 57 remained under treatment. By 1805 there were 220 admissions, 2,874 out-patients and 53 deaths; there were 1,286 vaccinations (p. 177). The bulk of the patients were destitute paupers sent in by the police, and more than half had wounds and other injuries. Twenty-one had ulcers and sores but infectious diseases were quite low – there was no cholera. There were very few surgical operations. Venereal disease was also low but special Lock-hospitals were well-established by 1811.

The Native Hospital at Benares opened in 1811, and the Calcutta Lying-in Hospital in 1814. In 1838 a small hospital was built in relation to the new Medical School in Calcutta (p. 199). When it was replaced by the new large hospital in 1853 this always admitted both Europeans and Indians. In Bombay, by 1809, there was a Native Hospital, supported by Government, with about 20 patients every day. In 1824 new hospitals were built for both the garrison and the civilian population. Additional native dispensaries were set up in 1834 and 1846, and a number of large hospitals were endowed as charities by wealthy Indians – in contrast to the other Presidency towns. In Madras in 1787 John Underwood, a Company surgeon, managed to get a piece of land for 'the indigent poor', and put up a building, the cost being met by voluntary subscription. There was a detached ward for brahmins, 'who, it was at first thought, would be reluctant to attend'. It was soon crowded, and patients were being turned away for lack of space. Two years later the Medical Board took control, paying rent and repairs as well as Underwood's salary as Attending Surgeon. By 1809 this had become the Native Hospital.

In the 1830s and 40s the first *mofussil* (provincial) civilian hospitals were founded by energetic Company surgeons who collected money, and gave their services free as this was not part of their duties. The building might be rented to the Company but remained the property of the surgeon's family for several generations, being run as a family business. This was commonly the case with the early lunatic asylums (p. 162). All hospitals were supplied with European medicines from the Company stores. By 1842 there were six hospitals in the Presidency outside Madras. In 1842 the main hospital in Madras was half for European military and half for European civilians. In the same enclosure was accommodation for European women and children, and Indians of both sexes in separate wards.

In 1785 General Sepoy Hospitals were replaced by individual Regimental Hospitals which were much preferred by the sepoys. The official Company staffing was one European assistant and one 'Black Doctor'[17] to each battalion. Their medical officers were convinced that these hospitals were more necessary for Indian soldiers than for European. The regimental medical officer got to know his men well, and could therefore detect 'fictitious complaints' better than the Head Surgeon at a General Hospital. There was continuing debate about the relation of General Hospitals to Regimental Hospitals. The sepoys preferred to remain in the care of colleagues of their own caste. But facilities at the Regimental Hospitals were necessarily limited, and their medical officers were repeatedly requested to send the more seriously ill patients to the General Hospital, including 'all Fluxes, fevers, Ulcerated Legs and Lues [venereal]'. They were criticized for holding on too long to their patients and so reducing their chances of recovery. But if too many were sent to the General Hospital, the facilities at the Regimental Hospitals would suffer. The medical officer might then have to send the sepoys to the Hospital with trivial complaints. In all cases the Medical Board required the regimental medical officers to follow their patients into the General Hospital and so gain extra experience.

The Native Doctor in each battalion supplied the sick with bazaar medicines 'at their own Cost'. If the (European) Assistant Surgeon thought that the patient could not be treated satisfactorily in this way, he was allowed to draw European medicines for him. The Native Doctors accompanied their regiments on service overseas, and were commended:

> ... on the last expedition, the Marine Battalion having returned, without the loss of a single man by sickness.

Among the requests to Madras from the Army in the Dekkan in 1806 was one for:

> two or three Sub-assistants [dressers] – one of those with careful looking after would be of more use than half a dozen Griffins.[18]

From 1806 the establishment was one dresser to each regiment of Indian cavalry, and two to each battalion of Indian infantry. Dressers were required to be 'natives of caste and respectability'. All applicants were examined by the medical officers in charge before being enrolled in a particular corps. Earlier they had been trained partly by individual surgeons and partly in hospital, but now all training was in General Hospitals as apothecaries, dressers and nursing attendants. Increasing importance was attached to general cleanliness and hygiene in the hospitals, with the patients being moved and cleaned regularly. There were many tributes to the skill and good service of the Indian nursing attendants,

> who are mostly brought up from an early period of their Lives, in these occupations, and habituated to the different dispositions of Sick Men, under various states of excruciating pain and affliction, which must naturally tend to ruffle the most temperate and placid mind. In these situations Hospital Servants are the more capable of rendering the Sick, wounded, and helpless patients, the most salutary comfort, by adapting themselves to the fretful and peevish turns of Patients, which long and painful illness must naturally induce.

Large numbers of Indians were employed in the hospitals, not only as nurses (one for every six men, and a separate nurse for a very ill patient when ordered by the Head Surgeon) and apothecaries, preparing and distributing medicines, but decoction-boilers, dooley-bearers, lint scrapers, 'biggaries' to powder medicines, water-men, cooks, boys for the wards, and messengers. Sepoy Hospitals needed a larger number of attendants of different castes as each caste would only carry out one duty. At the General Hospital in Madras the privies were often in need of repair, and there were complaints from the surgeons of the risks to the patients. It was necessary to recruit more 'totties' to empty the pots and wash them in the river every morning, but it was difficult to get enough men of a caste prepared to do this menial work.

By 1802 there were three large General Hospitals for Europeans in the Bombay Presidency, seven in Madras and six in Bengal. They were dependent on the regular supply of drugs and instruments from England, but the delay and loss en route led to over-indenting by the surgeons. Landing cargo at Madras was still hazardous. The ships had to anchor outside the surf and the cargo was carried in small boats. When the surf was too high 'the flag-staff is struck, as a signal that no insurance is payable on account of such losses as may happen'. The equipment might be useless. In 1792 portable cases of 'Capital Instruments' were distributed for trial on active service. But, although light to transport, the shortness of the knife and the smallness of the saw made them quite unsuitable for major amputations.

There were reprimands from the Directors for extravagances such as oatmeal for feeding the sick: 'the oatmeal is generally spoiled ... as it cannot reach India till it is at least one year old.' Surgeons were advised to use 'fresh Rice or other Grain which can always be procured on the spot', from which 'Gruel, equally good for Sick people can be prepared'. Only enough 'Vegetable Medicines' to last a year should be ordered, or, better still, replaced by 'the herbs of the Country which you can procure fresh'. The Apothecary was responsible for buying these bazar or 'country' medicines. He submitted his accounts each month on which he received 15 per cent commission. A list of bazar materials in 1789 included: limes, oranges, firewood, charcoal, material for poultices and fomentation, eggs, toddy, plantain leaves, butter, garlic, sugar, leather, cloth and lint for bandages, as well as medicines: quicksilver, opium, nitre, gum arabic, aloes, alum, asafoetida, camphor, liquorice root, cinnamon, nutmegs, cloves etc.

In 1795 the Directors asked Dr. John Hunter[19] to investigate the medical supplies of the Company. He found that there were many demands for medicines that had long gone out of use, as better ones had been discovered. The older preparations were less effective and more expensive. Salt of wormwood,

> made from the ashes of that plant was supposed to possess its peculiar virtues.[20] But improvements in Chemistry have taught us that the Salt procured from all wood ashes is the same, and it is an useless expense to prepare it from Wormwood, for if made from that Plant, it costs three times the price the other does when prepared agreeably to the directions of the College of Physicians.

Hunter recommended that prescriptions should conform to the Pharmacopoeias of the London and Edinburgh Colleges of Physicians. These were extensive enough to show that he did not wish to 'confine the Medical Servants within too narrow limits, and they can ask for others if they give good reasons'. New medicines were continually being assessed in London before the news could reach India, and Hunter proposed that good new remedies should be sent out to India without waiting for indents. He gave as an example a new species of Peruvian Bark — Yellow Bark — which had proved very valuable, and was 'cheaper and fresher than the Common Peruvian Bark now in the market'.

Up till now, insane Europeans had been housed in the prisons, often fettered. It was considered that insanity in India was more sudden and violent as a result of the climate; mechanical restraint was continued longer than in England. Any who could be restored to a reasonable state of health were sent back to England. As part of the lunacy reforms of the time, individual

Company surgeons began to collect money for separate buildings in which they gave their services free. The building might be rented to the Company but remained the property of the surgeon's family, being run as a family business. In Calcutta, by 1787, one surgeon had four patients in his own house which he had enlarged. In 1789 a separate Insane Hospital was opened with space for 11 officers and 22 soldiers, with Invalid Soldiers (pensioners) as attendants. In Madras, in 1794, there was a specially built house with 16 separate rooms with 'all necessary comforts and proper attendants'. In 1807 it was sold to James Dalton and for many years it was known as 'Dalton's Madhouse'. It remained in his family until the new Asylum was built in 1871. In Bombay an Asylum was built in 1826.

All the Lunatic Hospitals proved very expensive, and the Directors asked whether any individual benefit had been derived. In general it was cheaper to send the patients back to England as soon as possible, but they still had to be housed and treated until they were fit to travel. It was recognized that there was a much higher rate of cure in England, and the Directors arranged for soldiers, sailors and other servants of the Company to be treated in a private asylum in London.

A Hospital for Insane Native Soldiers was set up in Calcutta in 1798. Concern with acts of violence by insane civilian Indians led, in 1802, to the decision to set up asylums for both the criminal and the freely wandering insane in Bengal. Similar arrangements followed in Madras and Bombay. By 1820 there were six asylums in Bengal, four in Madras and one in Bombay. These were exclusively for Indians. The treatment followed the recommendations of the Select Committee on the madhouses in England (1815/16) 'rather than the traditions of yunani and ayurveda so easily at hand in India'. The patients, who were fed at Government expense, remained healthier than the ordinary prisoners who received a much smaller allowance and were subjected to hard labour. There was debate on the possibility that insanity was more easily curable in Indians than Europeans. Indians were more easily managed because of their habit of smoking ganja (cannabis) which was thought to be the cause of the insanity in nearly half the cases. In Europeans, alcohol was responsible for much of the violent insanity and for the deaths. Deaths in Indian lunatics were mostly due to fevers and dysentery.

A number of other special hospitals were set up: leper hospitals in Madras (1816) and Bombay (1890); eye hospitals in Bombay (1823) and Madras (1824). Lock-hospitals (venereal diseases) were well established in all areas by 1811. In 1789 the first special hospital for infectious diseases was set up for smallpox at Tellicherri.

The importance of a period of convalescence after serious illness was always recognized. There were places near the main settlements where the conditions were thought to be restorative, but no-one had much faith in them. Often the only course that seemed to hold out any hope was to get away from India on a sea voyage or return to England, but there was no home leave before 1764. The Cape of Good Hope was the next best, and the Company set up a 'sanitarium' there for civil and military officers. The new settlements in Australia were now also being recommended. The Swan River area (settled in 1829) had the advantage of the relatively short distance from India (25-30 days from Madras). Even better was Van Diemen's Land where everything was as in England. Everything tropical was left behind – surely the best of 'moral remedies for chronic disease'. If all convalescents could be sent to Hobart,

> it would certainly save vast numbers from death, or being invalided or discharged and sent home as unfit for further service in India.

Notes

1 The Boston Tea Party, December 1773.

2 This was the start of what would become the Indian Civil Service.

3 John Glass was appointed Assistant Surgeon at Bhagalpur in 1761 and remained there until 1815. He had two indigo factories.

4 Governor of Bombay (1798-1811). He had good relations with Indians, and was responsible for the reduction of infanticide (of girls) in Gujerat.

5 Leprosy. At this time leprosy was still confused with elephantiasis, and known to Jones and others as elephantiasis Graecorum (p. 100 f.n.16).

6 *munshi*, teacher, interpreter (Hind.).

7 *zamin-dar*, land-holder (Pers.)

8 Lord Hardinge was Governor-General from 1844-48; his grandson was Viceroy from 1910-16.

9 Rs. 100,000 = £12,500.

10 James Johnson, Surgeon in the Royal Navy, with fifteen years' experience in the East, wrote a textbook on tropical diseases in 1815 that was hardly changed in the sixth edition in 1841.

11 Increasing demand for European medicine from middle-class and wealthy Indians only started towards the end of the nineteenth century.

12 The zealot was suspended from a vertical pole by a rope attached to a metal hook through the tissues of his back, and he was then swung round.

13 'the Company's thieves look like bridegrooms'.

14 When committing suicide a Hindu would not hang himself in case his soul would be defiled by leaving through an impure channel, and he would rather throw himself over a cliff, drown or starve to death.

15 'Huts of mud and thatch house the bulk of the population of Calcutta, and a thousand people could have been accommodated in this way, whereas houses of masonry and timber, as the Europeans build for themselves, would only serve fifty'.

16 Gambling was long-established in India, although suppressed by the Muslims.

17 In 1802 the appointment of 'Black Doctors' was discontinued; those qualified were appointed as 'Dressers'.

18 Inexperienced newcomers to India (orig. unknown).

19 Examining Physician to the Company in London. The more famous John Hunter, the surgeon/anatomist, died in 1793.

20 Indian physicians had always attached great importance to the source of the wood ash for its specific medical properties, and they continued to do so.

Chapter Eleven
Renewed interest in Indian Medicine

For the greater part of the eighteenth century Europeans had looked scornfully at the 'unscientific' methods of Indian practitioners, but there was now an increasing interest in Indian Medicine and a desire to learn from its practitioners. Classical Indian Medicine, both Hindu and Muslim, was based on a written tradition, with principles that were similar to the humoral systems current in Europe up to the middle of the seventeenth century (p.13) and to some of the theories in vogue in the eighteenth century (p. 149). The British made little attempt to study Muslim (Unani) medicine at this time. With its decline under increasing Islamic orthodoxy (p. 14),

> the sciences were by no means encouraged, medicine, or rather quackery, alone was rewarded by moormen, hence pretenders to this science, makers of nostrums and provocatives, and sorcerers, are to be found in abundance wherever the Mahometan religion is established.

They concentrated on Ayurveda, trying to sift out anything of value for treating disease.

> Their practical principles are very similar to our own; and even their theories may be reconciled with ours, if we make allowance for their ignorance of anatomy, and the imperfection of their physiological speculations.

But folk-medicine, widespread in both Hindu and Muslim communities, was still not clearly distinguished from the classical systems. When the value of Indian Medicine was debated, depending on which system they encountered, the British regarded Indian physicians either as 'a set of ignorant cheats' or as 'miracles of knowledge and wisdom'. Surgeons at country stations where folk-medicine predominated saw most Indian practitioners as 'illiterate pretenders to knowledge ... quacks and vendors of nostrums'; if they had any texts, these were very garbled. Around Madras,

> the practitioners are poor men of a particular caste, who sit by the side of the high roads and market paths, with small boxes,

containing various kinds of powder, which is administered with particular instructions, and a promise of cure in a specific number of days.

For all complaints they insisted on abstinence, allowing the patient only rice gruel. Their remedies, which had been handed down unchanged from father to son for generations, included cinnabar (mercuric sulphide), used sometimes with success but often, by misuse, spreading ulceration further. They did not ask Europeans for help unless the case seemed hopeless. Men and women anointed their bodies with oil of sesamum which blocked the pores, and was used by the poor in winter instead of clothes. They recommended the principle for fevers – covering the whole body with a thick plaster of pounded herbs. The British regarded it as dangerous to close too many pores at one time, but this regime was cooling which they agreed with.

Folk-practitioners never bled their patients, but used the juice of the milk-bush[1] to raise a blister. There were no surgical operations, but they often applied the actual cautery, so that it was common to see horses, oxen and labourers, especially palanquin bearers and porters, with scars in various places. Fractures and dislocations were treated by the potters,[2] by putting the limb back into position and covering it with clay which acted as a splint when dry. But this often left the patients with deformed and stiff joints.

The preponderance of folk-practitioners tended to bias the British against Indian Medicine, but the surgeons were now trying to establish the value of Ayurveda compared with western medicine in the diagnosis and treatment of disease. In studying Indian diseases, some of them not well understood, the obvious course was to consult the local practitioners who, with their greater experience, might be expected to provide them with new and useful knowledge. Leprosy was a good example; it was 'a disease whose nature, classification, and treatment were not established'. India provided a wide field for study; Europe was hindered by lack of cases. In 1823 H. H. Wilson[3] discussed this in a paper on '*Kushta,* or Leprosy, as known to the Hindus' to the Medical and Physical Society of Calcutta. His first point was that all Hindu writers simply repeated the classical authors; there were no treatises on individual diseases. But their ideas on the causes of leprosy corresponded fairly well with the European, and they distinguished leprosy from other similar diseases which were often confused by experienced practitioners. Their treatment was 'essentially deficient'. They used multiple ingredients, which they claimed increased efficacy; many of these were 'preposterous and ridiculous'. But, however absurd when blended, some of the ingredients separately might prove useful, even if only as a palliative. Wilson recognized that some of the local preparations had active properties,[4] and he recommended their investigation to the members of the Society.

The Company had always urged its servants in country districts to look out for any native product that might be useful medicinally. Reports by medical and political officers on their districts usually included details of local diseases and the remedies used. Now it became official policy to require surgeons to note any medical treatment by an Indian that might be effective, and to collect the necessary drugs and herbs so that these could be sent in to the General Hospitals for clinical trial. If this was successful, the results would be published and circulated. If anything strange or unknown occurred in medical or veterinary practice, no treatment was to be undertaken until the local practitioners had been consulted and the local remedy evaluated. A number of Hindu remedies were found to be very effective, e.g. as purges and, particularly, for fevers, some of which, such as the kernel of the pod of 'cow-itch',[5] were nearly as powerful as Peruvian bark.

Renewed interest in Indian Medicine persuaded some Europeans to consult local practitioners. But over-enthusiasm for Indian methods was still suspect. An article in *Asiatick Researches* had stated that many hundreds of medicinal plants were unknown to, or wrongly described by, European botanists, but the author's remarks were received with caution, 'from the consideration of his avowed partiality towards native physicians'. There were also complaints by Company surgeons of the need to rescue patients who had too enthusiastically adopted Indian methods. One young man suffered a rapidly fatal illness after copying the Indian practice of eating hailstones.[6]

But the news of any successful treatment was spread by grateful patients. One man was relieved of a tape-worm 36 feet long, by a remedy which he had bought from a 'Mussulman fakeer'. The secret ingredient came from the stem of the pomegranate, and the prescription was published for general information. Among many other remedies there was a poultice of leaves, often prepared by palanquin bearers, for stubborn boils, which was successful in one or two days, where normally it would have taken eight to ten, and an ointment for 'ophthalmia' which relieved the pain when European treatment brought no relief. One of the most successful Indian treatments was the cooling of fevers, the 'refrigeration principle', which had been routinely adopted by the British (p. 87).

Europeans were surprised by the number of bath-houses in India. Hindus carried out their own 'fastidious ablutions', and the bath-houses were used mostly by Muslims and other races. The British were at first suspicious, feeling that such an indulgence would lead to weakening of the fibres. But they were convinced by the comfort of regular bathing in the heat, and even recognized that there were medical benefits. It was the same with the 'shampooing' (massage) that went with the baths – at first regarded as decadent, it was found to be 'soothing and therapeutic'. Hot bathing was regularly recommended for patients in hospital, and firewood and attendants became 'a necessary appendage of an Hospital'. When the supply of tin baths ran out, arrack casks were used.

Part of the reason for the enthusiasm for Indian Medicine was that some British surgeons continued to have faith in vigorous treatment, even as it became clear that this might be harmful in the tropics.[7] Bleeding *ad deliquium* [to syncope] was still sometimes recommended to check disease. But it was recognized that this itself could have serious complications, and leeches or blisters should be used instead.

But Hindu practitioners were criticized for being largely self-taught, without proper textbooks, and with no teaching institutions. They also relied on astrological calculations for the best times for collecting their herbs and for mixing and administering them. Sir William Jones had urged a study of their medicinal plants, noting that there were many hundreds of these, and that they were described in the classical texts. But this was countered by the view that, although Hindu practitioners might know the properties of their drugs, their total ignorance of physiology and pathology meant that they were applying one preparation to all stages of a disease and for diseases that might be quite different in nature. Their preparations were made up of multiple ingredients. If it was difficult to assess the result of a single drug, how much more so with a mixture of many herbs and minerals. The argument was not about the merits of many of the drugs in use, but about the competence of the practitioners to evaluate them.

It was generally held that very little surgery was being practised by Indians. But the British now discovered that some traditional techniques persisted in scattered families where a particular craft had been handed down from father to son, often in conditions of great secrecy. The status of surgery established by Susruta had steadily declined, so that these practitioners were all from the lower castes (p. 11). It is perhaps surprising that so little was known of these craft operations until the end of the eighteenth century. But, like folk-medicine everywhere, the techniques remained closely-guarded family secrets for fear of financial loss and that any remedies would lose their efficacy if they became public knowledge. This was also a time when the British were actively looking for Indian remedies, and communication between practitioners was encouraged by the authorities.

Three of these techniques caught the attention of British surgeons: cutting for stone, couching for cataract, and grafting skin for mutilations of the face. These had all been described by Susruta, and the techniques of the first two had been handed down unchanged. The third had become a tradition with the *koomars* or potters.[8] The principle of the operation of grafting a flap of skin and subcutaneous tissue remained, but the technique had been altered by taking this from the forehead (p. 171) and not from the cheek.

The technique of cutting for stone was the 'low lithotomy' – the 'lesser' operation or the 'apparatus minor' – through an incision in the perineum, using a knife and hook only (p. 9). There were some successful cases, witnessed by European surgeons. But many of the Indian lithotomists, who claimed a high success rate, did not keep a register and left the stones in situ. They would only operate on favourable cases, and then only after an application to the authorities to ensure that they would not be prosecuted if the patient died.

The cataract operation by 'couching' (p. 10) was becoming obsolete by European standards. But some Company surgeons considered that the technique described by Susruta was still practicable, and could be taught to Indians for use in areas where no European was available. But others, seeing the work of the travelling cataract surgeons, reported that some of the operations were fraudulent – the practitioner claiming to have shifted the lens when it still remained in place. Many others resulted in irreparably damaged eyes. In general, the high rate of complications led to its gradual abandonment and replacement by techniques introduced from Europe.

But in skin grafting for mutilations of the face, particularly the reconstruction of the nose with skin from the forehead, the potters showed great skill. Their technique was studied and practised by Company surgeons. Their reports, transmitted to England in 1794, had a major influence on the development of surgery in Europe (p. 173).

Indians also carried out some minor operations, mostly using the cautery or caustics to deal with small tumours, or threads medicated with caustic paste to heal sinuses and fistulae as described by Susruta (p. 10). Some of these techniques were successful, but others left deep scars. If the lesion was large, it was regarded as unsuitable for treatment, and the patients either came directly, or were referred, to the nearest British hospital.

Early travellers in India, e.g. the Dutchman van Linschoten (p. 26), had recorded that adultery was punished by cutting off the nose – usually as a private act of revenge. But it was also a judicial punishment. In South India, minor offences were punished by cutting off the nose and ears, and adultery by a man by cutting off his nose. Cutting off the nose was also the standard treatment for prisoners of war. In the war of the Emperor Aurangzeb against Bijapur in 1686, the men of Bijapur cut off the noses of any of the Mogul's men that they captured. Tippoo Singh in the Third Mysore War (1792) cut off the noses and right hands of his prisoners. Loss of the nose was not only very unsightly, but it was the stigma of a criminal or prisoner of war. There were good reasons for the victims to seek reconstruction, and the few families with the necessary skills were much sought after.

The classical operation of Susruta used flaps of skin from the cheeks to repair defects of the nose, lips or ears. Since the amount of skin available is limited, only relatively small defects could be repaired. The technique of the potters that attracted the attention of British surgeons used flaps from the much larger area of skin of the forehead.⁹

Operations similar to Susruta's were carried out in Europe from the early fifteenth century, but there is nothing resembling the 'Indian' method. It is not known when the technique changed from one to the other in India, although the potters' method has been traced back to a number of families in the Deccan in the sixteenth century. When Company surgeons questioned the Indian practitioners at the end of the eighteenth century they were told that the operation had been passed down in their families from 'time immemorial'.¹⁰

The first description by a European of this 'Indian' operation is by Niccolao Manucci, one of the Venetian adventurers in India in the seventeenth century. He saw the Mogul's soldiers who had been captured and mutilated by the men of Bijapur in the war of 1686:

> thus they came back into the camp all bleeding. The surgeons belonging to the country cut the skin of the forehead above the eyebrows, and made it fall down over the wounds on the nose. Then, giving it a twist so that the live flesh might meet the other live surface, by healing applications they fashioned for them other imperfect noses ... I saw many persons with such noses, and they were not so disfigured as they would have been without any nose at all, but they bore between their eyebrows the mark of the incision.

The first European to use this technique, which he had copied from local practitioners, was the Company surgeon Lucas¹¹ in Madras. He carried out several of these operations successfully – probably at some time before 1782. A similar operation, by a potter, was witnessed in Poona in March 1793 by two Company surgeons of the Bombay Presidency, Thomas Cruso and James Findlay. They had never seen, nor indeed heard of, such an operation. Apparently they did not know of Lucas's operations which were never published. The patient, a Mahratta of the caste of husbandman, had been employed as a bullock-driver in the Company Army in the Third Mysore War (1792). He had been taken prisoner by Tippoo Singh's men, and had had his nose and his right hand cut off. At the end of the war he was returned to the British and became a pensioner of the Company in Poona. The British had a number of similarly mutilated pensioners, and they were alerted to the possibility of reconstruction by an itinerant salesman with a scar on his forehead. When questioned, he told them that he had been convicted of adultery, and that his nose had been amputated by the public executioner. The reconstruction had been carried out by a potter. This 'surgeon' was sent for, and he reconstructed the noses of five pensioners.[12] He said that he could also repair defects of the lips.

The two Company surgeons recorded the details, and had illustrations made. Their account was sent to England and published in October 1794 as a letter to *The Gentleman's Magazine*:

> A friend has transmitted to me the following very curious, and, in Europe, I believe, unknown chirurgical operation, which has long been practised in India with success; namely, affixing a new nose on a man's face.

The letter was accompanied by a reproduction of a copper-plate engraving that had been made in Bombay, showing the patient ten months after the operation. The British surgeons had questioned the Indian about his training, and he had told them that he learned the technique from his father, and he from his father.

Their report attracted attention in Europe and America. In London the surgeon Joseph Constantine Carpue collected and published all the available information. He had to wait until 1814 before a suitable patient presented for the operation. On 23 October he carried out the first 'Indian' operation in Europe, and published two successful cases in 1816. Both patients were army officers – the first nose had been destroyed by over-dosage with mercury for a liver complaint, and the second by a sabre cut in battle. Carpue was followed, in 1817, by von Graefe, the professor of surgery in Berlin. The operation was then taken up by other surgeons in Europe and America, and it was the starting-point of the modern specialty of plastic and reconstructive surgery.

British surgeons in India in the second half of the nineteenth century were often required to carry out these reconstructions, and they used either the classical or the 'Indian' method, as appropriate. The scar on the forehead from which the graft was taken was an additional disfigurement in a European, but in Indians it could be hidden by the turban. The surgeons commented on the frequency of nasal mutilation, and on their consequent experience of reconstruction, which was far greater than that of contemporary surgeons in Europe. Although there were many cases of nasal destruction in Europe, these were very often due to syphilis. Since the disease was often incompletely cured, the remaining infected tissues provided a poor bed for the reception of a skin flap, and reconstruction was often unsuccessful.

In the early eighteenth century the British had noted the long-standing Indian technique of inoculation (the live virus) for **smallpox** (p. 91). They were to be responsible for the introduction of vaccination (cowpox) which was much safer and more effective. But this was not developed in England until

1798, and brought to India in 1802. Faced with epidemic smallpox in India they set up inoculation programmes from about 1785. There was a strong tradition of inoculation in Bengal but there was resistance in other parts of India. This was being overcome when vaccination was started, arousing further opposition. The British had to struggle for several years before it was established.

Smallpox commonly appeared after the rainy season, i.e. from December for several months. It was most fatal in February, March and April, becoming milder with the hot weather and disappearing in June. In open country, where there were no endemic fevers, it was the major epidemic. In Bengal an epidemic kept the gardeners busy; the physicians retired, a gardener was summoned, and elaborate ceremonies were carried out. Inoculation was believed to have originated in Bengal, and to be confined to Hindus. Vaidyas never inoculated, regarding blood and pus as pollution. Muslims had religious prejudices against it. The inoculators (**tikadars**) came from a particular lower order of brahmins. They travelled in circuits, timed to arrive several weeks before the disease was expected – in Bengal, early in February. Some stayed in the cities, others went out into the country. On an auspicious day in February/April they inoculated the children, charging according to the means of the families. Their technique was well-established, as reported by Joseph Holwell in 1767 (p. 108). They never used fresh matter, but a cloth impregnated from the previous year, moistened with Ganges water. After the operation they insisted on a careful regime of light diet, cooling and fresh air. They realized that inoculation carried a high risk of starting an outbreak of smallpox. In a closed community, such as village or a ship, the risk could be reduced by inoculating the whole community. They always tried to inoculate all the inhabitants of a village at the same time. In isolated districts and among the hill people inoculation might be carried out by the lowest castes, making a crude incision and rubbing the matter in with a finger. Some of these primitive tribes showed relatively few of their number marked with smallpox. Some hill tribes were regarded as savages, but, by good treatment, they could be 'persuaded to inoculation'. One landholder sent his own doctor into the Garrow Hills in an epidemic. After that,

> they provided themselves yearly with an inoculator, whom they reward in the most liberal manner, and take as much care of, while he resides among them, as if he were their father.

Europeans in India were in general prejudiced against inoculation for the greater part of the eighteenth century; in an epidemic they fled to the country. The first inoculations by the British, from about 1785, were on British soldiers and their families; most were successful, but there were some deaths. In 1786 all the children in the charge of the Orphan Society in Calcutta who had not had smallpox were inoculated. The 53 who were inoculated all recovered, but there were three deaths among the nine children who caught the natural disease. In 1794 the Madras Government suggested that boys from the Male Orphan Asylum, who were to be inoculated, should be sent in to the General Hospital for the period required by the standard regimen. But the Medical Board objected because of the danger that they would start an epidemic and infect the patients already in the hospital.

For the soldiers there was no compulsion for inoculation, and the decision was left to each man. But for those who were willing, winter was regarded as the best time, and General Orders were issued to the Army that 'the Surgeons of Stations and Corps do promote, as much as possible, the practice of Inoculation amongst all description of persons'. It was more difficult to convince the sepoys than the British soldiers but they began to come forward and bring their children. Inoculations were carried out by the medical officers in public, and with great ceremony, to convince the spectators of the simplicity of the operation.

But inoculation of the civilian population made slow progress in some parts of the country. Indian inoculators were most common in Bengal. The local people had become accustomed to them over a long period, and were aware of the benefits. Conditions were quite different in south India, and there was great resistance from the villagers.

> No argument could prevail against those rooted Prejudices against the Customs of Europe, imbibed by the natives from their earliest infancy, and cherished with a blind enthusiasm throughout their mature years.

The Head Surgeon at Trichinopoly was commended for inoculating 86 local inhabitants. He had started with the Portuguese padres, and when that was a success they went round recommending it to all their parishioners. He completed 225 inoculations without a casualty, and believed that he had 'done away the prejudices of the Natives'. Government ordered that this success should be given public notice 'to encourage the other medical gentlemen'.

Europeans were now more in favour of inoculation, 'and it is only the native inhabitants that demand our further attention'. Collectors were authorized to employ and pay extra brahmin doctors as inoculators, 'so as to ensure a general inoculation next cold season'. In Madras it was, at first, the policy to reward those who came to be inoculated, and this had been helpful in overcoming local prejudice. But it was seen that 'by encouraging resistance to the practice on any other terms it is calculated to frustrate the permanent establishment of the measure'. There would be better results from training 'a few intelligent Bramin doctors in each District to become practitioners of inoculation by applying to their interests as well as their prejudices'. Their interests were to be ensured by payment according to the numbers treated. The authorities were even prepared to give financial support to Indian religious ceremonies if these would help to overcome opposition by 'propitiating the deity who is supposed to preside over this dreadful Malady' (p. 91). Individual surgeons then started training Indian inoculators. At first this was only on a small scale and in one or two villages. But the inhabitants were beginning to lose their fear of inoculation, and now the villagers mixed in the crowd with the patients under inoculation.

Edward Jenner's first observations on cowpox had been made in 1768 but the results were not published until 1798. The advantages of cowpox vaccination over smallpox inoculation were then so quickly established in Europe that inoculation programmes in India were postponed to wait for sufficient supplies of lymph to arrive. Most European countries tried to discourage inoculation. In India the Government legislated against it. It was banned in Bengal in 1802-3 on the report by the Superintendent General of Vaccine Inoculation that the mortality was 1 in 200 Indians, and 1 in 60-70 Europeans in Calcutta, as a result of spreading infection. Much of the resistance came from the brahmin inoculators who would lose their livelihood. Some were convicted and heavily fined. But in 1831 there were still 10-15 inoculators in Calcutta. Their activities meant that smallpox was kept alive in the city, from where it spread to every part of Bengal. There was no possibility of eradicating the disease until they were prohibited. Some of them were persuaded to train as vaccinators. But the custom was difficult to suppress, and it continued on a limited scale into the twentieth century.

When lymph for vaccination reached India in June 1802 'on the points of ivory lancets contained in hermetically sealed glass phials' it had been obtained from cows in Lombardy, and despatched via Vienna to Baghdad.[13] A vaccinated child from Baghdad was sent to Basra, and this material was continued in a weekly succession of patients, and so by stages to Bombay. The first successful vaccination in India (14 June 1802) was on the three-year-old daughter of an Anglo-Indian servant of a British army officer. Within four months there were more than 1000 vaccinations in Bombay. It was then introduced into other parts of India. Attempts to transmit the vaccine to Bengal failed, until Dr Anderson in Madras vaccinated a boy of thirteen, and sent him by sea. On the voyage the virus was kept alive through a chain of children (mostly Anglo-Indian and low-caste boys) until it reached Calcutta on 17 November 1802 on both arms of a boy of fifteen. Through him vaccination was established in Bengal. Within the first few months nearly all the European children had been vaccinated, and surgeons in outlying stations and army units then took up the practice. But fresh material was often difficult to maintain, particularly in the hot seasons, and supplies had to be sent out from central depots.[14] However, 11,166 vaccinations were carried out in the first eighteen months, 'a matter of great importance, when it is considered, that, in India, at least one in sixty dies of those inoculated with the smallpox'.

As the success of vaccination became clear, there were claims by brahmins that it had been known in India in much earlier times. An ancient Sanskrit book was cited as the authority. There was also an account by a nobleman of Benares of his son, ill with smallpox, and the brahmin who took threads soaked in matter from the pustule on a cow, and pulled it through the skin of both upper arms on needles. These and similar accounts were published in the *Asiatic Journal*, and so reached Europe where they were cited as authoritative. Investigations by surgeons and others in India, however, showed that the claims were false. The passage in the Sanskrit text was an interpolation, and the use of thread was a British method. Genuine cowpox did not occur in Indian cattle, and there was even great difficulty in keeping imported cowpox virus alive in the Indian climate. There was some evidence that deliberate attempts ('pious frauds') may have been made by British officials, by composing appropriate Sanskrit verses, to influence the brahmins to support vaccination. At the time, the authorities thought it was a great pity that the deception had been discovered, for nothing could have been a greater help in promoting vaccination than 'the testimony of such an ancient authority'. Instead of dismissing the book as another of the 'fraudulent claims of the Bramins to the prior possession of all kinds of science', it should have been accepted in view of the immense benefits that would result.

When they started to carry the vaccination programme into the country districts the British were astonished at the resistance they encountered. It was expected that Hindus would eagerly take to vaccination as the material came from the cow which was sacred. But villagers objected to the cow as a source of lymph. They were familiar with the diseases that caused a discharge from the tongue and feet of their cows, and they assumed that they were to be injected with similar material. They also had the idea that, if they were exempt from smallpox, their cattle would get it, or there might be an outbreak of cholera. Further, they believed

> it impious to have recourse to any means of averting this scourge, save offerings to their tutelary gods, and they esteem all endeavours to cure it dangerous, as tending to exasperate the Deity.

These objections were supported by the brahmin inoculators whose livelihood was threatened, and who now prevented the children from being brought forward. If the brahmins could not be persuaded, the introduction of vaccination would be impossible. Continuation of inoculation would lead to recurrent epidemics as the disease was regenerated annually.

Government action was to send out explanatory notices in all Indian languages to convince the chiefs and respected elders in the villages, and then to recruit Indian vaccinators. Missionaries were also urged to persuade their followers. A number of Indian families took up the profession of public vaccinator, handing on their skills to their sons. Bonuses were awarded according to the number of vaccinations that they carried out. They could also

> earn a considerable sum yearly by executing the Sitala worship, and when a child is vaccinated, a portion of the service is performed ... a curious compromise between the indigenous faith and European medical science.

Some of them were attacked by villagers,[15] suspicious that Government was trying to interfere with their religion, or that they were 'marking' children, particularly the boys who would then be sent as coolies to other British colonies or into the army, or that the mark was part of a census to impose a new tax.

But in some parts of the country the brahmins were persuaded to let their children be vaccinated, and the people followed their example. At first, vaccination was confined to the winter, to avoid the fevers of summer. The troops, including the sepoys, were always the first concern of the authorities. For indigent civilians, rice and food were provided during treatment as an inducement. Sheds were erected for those who had no houses, and to guard against spread of disease into the towns. There was no compulsion, and only those who were willing were treated at first. But it was the policy to try to persuade all the members of a community to be vaccinated at the same time. This was important in the early days, as there were occasional fatalities – usually from some unrelated cause, but enough to increase resistance to the programme. There was still some prejudice against European medical measures in the higher castes, and there was difficulty in gaining access to their women and children.

Reports of success began to come in from outlying districts. In Masulipatam the surgeon successfully vaccinated the child of a man of 'rank and opulence'. This was such an important example to the people that the surgeon asked permission to give the father a pair of pistols. The Governor of Madras, Lord Clive (son of Robert Clive), was an enthusiastic supporter of vaccination. He opened his garden as a Vaccination Centre, and guaranteed the supply of rice for the patients. There were problems with the potency of the vaccine, which was sent out from the centre by post, or on suitable subjects or children under the charge of a vaccinator, by ship if necessary. Before a voyage, the Captain was instructed that individuals were to be vaccinated in succession throughout the voyage.

Indian vaccinators were given an allowance for every hundred successful vaccinations; each of these had to be countersigned by the local British official. In the areas where they were well-known, the vaccinators had so many successful cases that it was felt that it might be necessary to limit the payment. It was noted that the Government allowance for a hundred vaccinations would allow the practitioner to live comfortably for several months. In the first eighteen months in Bengal 11,166 persons were vaccinated. Credit was given to the brahmins who had 'risen superior to prejudice', and whose powerful influence had persuaded all other castes of Hindus. The people in areas without a vaccinator began to petition Government that one should be provided. By 1806 the vaccination programme was fully established. In 1844 it was possible to write that, in some areas, 'smallpox is seldom heard of'.

As well as training Indian dressers and vaccinators, it was now official policy to encourage general education; this had been started in 1813 (p. 152). The General Committee of Public Instruction was appointed by Government in 1823 to suggest measures for 'the better instruction of the people'. More colleges and schools were to be set up for Indians to study in the vernaculars. Medicine was one of the subjects to be taught. Already in May 1822 a memorandum from the Medical Board had stressed the need for a Native Medical Institution for the education of Indian medical practitioners. This was agreed by Government, and the Institution opened in October 1824. Teaching was in Sanskrit at the Calcutta Sanskrit College (Hindu) and in Urdu at the Calcutta Madrassa (Muslim). European medical texts were translated into Sanskrit, Bengali and Urdu, and Company surgeons wrote special textbooks on diseases important in India. There were twenty students, selected by Superintending Surgeons.

The students received a small salary during training, and after qualifying, if they entered Government service, they were to serve the Army or Civil department as Sub-Assistant Surgeons for fifteen years. Most of the teachers were from the Company's medical service. The course was for three years, with pharmacy, physiology and anatomy in the first year, and medicine and surgery in the next two, with clinical training at the General Hospitals, Eye Infirmary, and the Department of Vaccination. Dissection of the human body was not carried out; there were some animal dissections, and the students attended post-mortems. At the Sanskrit College, Caraka, Susruta and other classical Hindu writers were studied, and Avicenna and the Arab physicians at the Madrassa. In 1826, the number of students was raised to fifty, and, in 1831, a small hospital with thirty beds was opened, attached to the Sanskrit College.

In Madras the organization of the subordinate establishment was set up in 1827. Europeans and Eurasians started as 'medical apprentices', and graduated to Apothecary. Indians started as 'medical pupils', and progressed to First Dresser. There were different rates of pay for the two branches. The course was mainly practical. The apprentices kept journals of the cases under their care, and gave out the medicines prepared by the candidates attached to the dispensary. They prepared diet sheets, and copied out the prescriptions written by the Assistant Surgeons. In dangerous diseases they were required to keep watch by the bedside, noting the progress of the patient between the visits of the medical officers; they were relieved every two hours. There was some theoretical instruction in anatomy and physiology, and they were taught to bleed, apply leeches and blisters, and dress sores of every description. After varying periods in a hospital, the surgeon of the hospital would put forward names to fill vacancies in the subordinate medical establishment.

From 1825-35 166 Indian doctors from the Institution in Calcutta, entered the public service. The best of them were taken on to the strength as Sub-Assistant Surgeons. This was the start of the formal medical training of Indians, resulting in the Civil Assistant Surgeon grade, of whom there were more than 500 in 1914.

The founding of these traditional schools was a further spur to Company surgeons to take an interest in Indian Medicine, and to review and produce editions of the classical texts on which a number of studies were then published. The exchange of ideas with Indian practitioners led to recommendations of Indian medicines for official use, particularly for the sepoys.

But the feeling that all education should be on western lines was growing. Dr. John Tytler, who had been appointed Superintendent of the Sanskrit College in 1830, was a distinguished Oriental scholar who had supported the view that Indians should be taught in their own languages. But he came to feel that this instruction was relatively rudimentary, and that the vernaculars did not lend themselves to advanced study of European texts.

Notes

1 *Euphorbia tirucalli*, 'milk-hedge', has an acrid milky juice, powerful enough to kill fish when thrown into running water.

2 Potters or tile-makers (koomar caste) also had a family tradition of operations to reconstruct missing parts of the face (p. 171).

3 Wilson had joined the Bengal Medical Service in 1808. He became Professor of Sanskrit at Oxford University.

4 For example, chaulmoogra oil and hydnocarpus oil (p. 222). Also arsenic, mercury and other metals 'treated according to the alchemical notions of the Hindus' (p. 12).

5 Cowage, *Macuna pruriens*,

6 Hailstones were rare in India, and were thought to have powerful medicinal virtues. In a hailstorm Indians would swallow as many as they could.

7 *Some doctors in India would make Plato smile;*
  If you fracture your skull they pronounce it the bile ...
  And with ointment mercurii and pills calomelli,
  They reduce all the bones in your skin to a jelly ...
  Broke down by the climate, low, weak, t'would surprise ye
  To hear them insist that your blood is too sizey. (1825)

8 The potters were commonly made fun of in their villages and in proverbs, and were generally regarded as rather stupid.

9 This has come to be known as the 'Indian' operation. It still has a place in reconstructive surgery today for defects not only of the nose but of other parts of the face.

10 The operation continued as a family craft throughout the nineteenth century, but now seems to have died out; all reconstructions are carried out by qualified surgeons.

11 Colley Lyon Lucas (1730-97) was in India continuously from 1762, becoming Surgeon-General to the Madras Army in the Second Mysore War.

12 He was always referred to afterwards as 'the artist of Poona'.

13 Jenner had sent lymph to India by sea in 1799 but the ship foundered at the Cape of Good Hope and never reached India.

14 The first lymph sent to China from Bombay in October 1803 lost its virulence on the voyage.

15 See 'The Tomb of his Ancestors' in *The Day's Work* (Kipling).

V
WESTERNIZATION (1835-58)

Chapter Twelve
Establishment of western ('modern') medicine

The Company continued to extend its area of influence. With the arrival of Lord Wellesley, the eldest of the three Wellesley brothers, as Governor-General in 1798, the policy of taking over the territories of weak Indian princes was intensified. In May 1799, after the fall of Seringapatam and the death of Tippoo, Mysore became a vassal state with Arthur Wellesley (later Duke of Wellington) as Governor. Where previously war had been justified to protect the Company's trading interests, a state of almost continuous war was now needed to protect its new territories. By 1820 the Company's armies were the largest in the world.

Lord Wellesley was severely criticized by the Company – 'the General fights, and the Company pays.' But the complaints by the Directors of the huge expenses were often disregarded by the increasingly powerful generals and governors in India. The local men felt, as before, that they were not being supported by the authorities at home who did not seem to appreciate the size of their conquests, or that the administrative arrangements suitable for a factory could not cope with a whole province.

In 1800, debts were accumulating in India, and there was general unrest, with large areas of central India over-run by the Mahrattas. Cornwallis was sent out again to restore order, but the Mahrattas were not finally controlled until the victories of Arthur Wellesley ended the Second Mahratta War in 1805. The First Burma War (1823-6) led to the occupation of Rangoon. There were disasters in the First Afghan War (1838-42), exacerbated by the rivalry between Company officers and Royal officers. The Sind War (1843) gave the Company control over the rich and fertile valley of the Indus. The Sikh Wars of 1845-6 and 1848-9 ended with the whole of the Punjab in British hands. All military action was still taken in the name of the Company, but there was more and more talk of 'British India' and the 'Empire', particularly by the Army.

With the rise of imperialism under the Wellesleys, the liberal influence of William Jones and the orientalists began to wane as they were outnumbered by the reformers who were becoming more arrogant and hostile to Indians.[1] To the reformers, secular and religious, India was 'imprisoned in authority, in custom and in tradition'. With the obvious loss of power of their rulers the whole nation was not only of inferior quality but incapable of improvement.

James Forbes, a firm evangelical, wrote in his memoirs of many years in India that

> a long and more intimate intercourse with the Brahmins and higher classes of Hindoos had rather lessened them in my esteem ... The lives of the luxurious priests, the ignorance of the worshippers, and the penances of the devotees, now appeared not only superstitious, but useless and absurd. The unhallowed fires were still kindled for the innocent female victims; the temples still open to the higher castes of Hindoos, still shut against the poor chandala [outcast] and humbled paria.

These views were encouraged in England by James Mill's (1817) influential book.[2] He criticized William Jones, and aimed to show the subordinate position of Indian culture and civilization, with recommendations for sweeping reforms. Mill had never been to India but his opinion carried great weight, and his book became required reading for the Company at home and for British administrators in India. It was generally held that nothing new could come out of India. The only course was thought to be the abandonment of Indian ways, and the development of education on western lines.

Lord (Thomas Babington) Macaulay, as Secretary of the Board of Control, had presented the Act to Parliament for the Company's new Charter of 1833. He then went to India for four years as President of the Committee of Public Instruction to promote the new educational policy, declaring that he would resign rather than continue an old system that 'did not accelerate the progress of truth but delayed the natural death of expiring errors'.[3] The policy was reinforced in 1835 by the adoption of English as the official language of India, as recommended by Macaulay. Successive Governor-Generals then acted to implement westernization by improving law and order. In 1829 Bentinck outlawed suttee in one of the first reforms of Hindu customs by legislation. Slavery was abolished in 1843, and there was a gradual reduction in child marriage and female infanticide. Under Dalhousie, from 1847, work started on the railway system, the telegraph, irrigation works, bridges, canals, roads, and the beginnings of elementary and secondary education.

This reversal of the earlier liberal attitude to Indian culture included Indian Medicine:

> When the British came to India, the efficiency of both these systems [Ayurveda and Unani] was at a low ebb, no improvements having taken place and no important discoveries having been made since the ancient treatises were

written. The study of Anatomy, the very ground-work of Surgical Science had fallen into disuse owing to superstitious injunctions. The treatment of diseases was necessarily empirical. No corresponding development of these Sciences took place in India during the decades in the nineteenth century when remarkable progress was taking place in the Western World.[4]

After 1835 there was no official support for Indian Medicine, and most Europeans became increasingly opposed to it. The Native Colleges that had been set up by the Company were closed to make way for teaching on purely western lines (p. 199). Teaching of Indian Medicine was confined almost entirely within the family. These practitioners were responsible for the treatment of the greater part of the population, particularly in rural areas. Their treatment was expensive, and, although the poor might prefer Indian Medicine, they often had to accept free treatment from the British. The middle and richer classes of Indians gradually came to make increasing demands for European medicine.

Sir William Jones had extolled the practitioners of classical Indian Medicine as 'the most virtuous and amiable of the Hindoos'. Some surgeons still regarded them favourably as 'doctors by long descent, well taught, and widely knowledgeable as well as correct, obliging, and communicative'; their defects might be recognized, but it should be possible to learn something from them, particularly in view of the esteem in which they were held by their educated countrymen. Others noted their 'barbarous empiricism', which 'takes advantage of ignorant credulity', but that their practice should be investigated to find anything that might be beneficial and to expose anything harmful.

Medical journals published Indian remedies that had been tried, and found to be effective. Some of the preparations were nearly as good as quinine for fevers. Some were better than the standard British drugs – a prescription for ring-worm was 'more effective and less painful'. Others drugs had active properties, but needed further research. Many of the Indian preparations could easily be obtained from local drug sellers, as they were all in general use. Some of these, such as croton oil, became popular in Europe. *Croton tiglium* had long been used by Indians. Now, prepared by the British as a tincture which allowed accurate dosage, it provided the strong purge necessary at the onset of a fever; it was an important preparation for the surgeon on campaign, for 500 doses of it could be 'contained in a small wafer-box, and purchased for half a rupee'. Indian drugs were generally cheaper than European, which were often kept for treating Europeans. When an Indian drug was found to be as effective as the European equivalent it was recommended for use in the Native Hospitals instead of expensive European drugs.

The preface to the first volume of the *Transactions of the medical and physical Society of Calcutta* (1825) stated that 'the materia medica of the East has long contributed to the pharmacy of Europe, and there is no reason to suppose that its stores are exhausted'. But it could not be expected that

> the imperfect science of the Baids or Hakeems of India, shall offer any instructive lessons to their better educated brethren of Europe.

The early journals in Calcutta and Bombay gave lists of Indian medicines, with occasional notes for their clinical use, and reports of those which had been tried, proved successful, and should be more widely known. Trials at the General Hospitals were carried out at the request of the Medical Societies, and on the command of the Medical Boards. Potentially useful preparations were handed out at medical meetings for experiment. It was noted that Indian practitioners usually combined the active ingredient with many other ingredients. There was always the problem of identifying the correct herb, and dealers might substitute inferior varieties; this was not necessarily due to chicanery, but often to ignorance. In the Hindu pharmacopoieas animal products were rare, compared with the very large number of vegetable, and many of them were rendered obsolete by the development of chemistry. Their continued use was mostly by peripatetic quacks, although it was noted that antelope horn, which was much favoured, was chemically the same as stag horn, which still had a place in the pharmacopoeias of London and Edinburgh. As formerly in Europe, Indians attached different properties to the ash of different plants (p. 162). But their habit of prescribing *Mithradates*[5] meant, that in order to reduce the bulk, 'they are obliged to subject many of their vegetable remedies to the action of fire'; thus they were administering potassium carbonate more often than they realized. It was sometimes difficult to get accurate information about Indian drugs from practitioners who might be unreliable in the identification, or unwilling to identify, fearing for their livelihood. Local people might be more reliable – they had less knowledge, but they were less deceitful.

Although some of the Indian drugs were of proven value, there were many criticisms of the medical system as a whole. Thomas Wise (a Company surgeon 1827-51), in his *Commentary* on Hindu medicine, described their doctrine of the causation of some diseases by numerous devils. He thought that this enabled the brahmins to account for many diseases that they did not understand, and allowed them to gain a rich living from their ignorant patients. Hakeems, also, had little knowledge of anatomy; their treatment of serious diseases was feeble, and their remedies 'inert, and sometimes worse'. Blindness in one or both eyes often followed their treatment of purulent ophthalmia. 'In surgery their notions are fully as crude and barbarous' – the only remedy for external bruising being to rub the part with turmeric and cow-dung.

In Europe, medicine and the basic sciences were each contributing to the other; many scientists of this period were physicians. Advances in chemistry meant that physiology was now the study of chemical reactions in the body; alchemy had long since been discredited. Homoeopathy had started as a regular part of medicine at the end of the eighteenth century, but criticism now restricted its use.[6] Analysis of standard drugs led to the isolation of the active principle, with greater effect and more certain dosage, e.g. morphine from opium, quinine from bark. Detailed studies of the pathology of disease, and the application of statistics to treatment, were showing the inefficacy of the old heroic measures. These advances were disseminated by the rapid increase in the number of medical and scientific societies and their journals.

In 1800 the Corporation of Surgeons became the Royal College of Surgeons of London, which issued diplomas for the right to practise surgery. In 1821 the Company introduced new regulations for candidates for its medical service. The age limit was raised to 'not under twenty years', and in 1836 to twenty-two. As well as a diploma from the College of Surgeons or one of the Scottish Colleges,[7] the candidate had to show a certificate of dexterity in the art of cupping, obtained from a public hospital in London, and of six months attendance at an approved general hospital. He also had to pass an examination by the Company's Examining Physician, and attend a course of lectures in Hindustani (Urdu). After 1835 no medical officer would be appointed until he had passed a colloquial examination in Hindustani, Mahratti or Gujarathi. From 1852 he had to provide certificates of attendance for three months at a Lunatic Asylum and proficiency in diseases of the eye. He had to pay his passage out, and, from 1828, take with him a copy of Annesley's *Sketches of the most prevalent Diseases of India*. The first competitive examinations were held in 1855, and were then only open to British candidates.

On arrival in India the new surgeon, as before, spent three months in a General Hospital where

> all our Medical men confess that upon their arrival here they
> are to study cases which are quite new to them, and a practice
> which they had never been acquainted with before.

After three months as Assistant Surgeon he would have to serve at least three years with the Army before being considered for any other post. Definitive medical texts were now available on the most prevalent diseases, medicinal plants and drugs, and Hindu materia medica. The Government provided funds for these, and took up copies for distribution to the Medical Service. Medical Societies were formed in Calcutta (1823) and Bombay (1835), and these produced regular volumes of *Transactions*.

The hazards of life in India were reflected in the life assurance premiums. In 1827 the premium was more than twice as much at age twenty-one, and one and a half times as much at fifty, as in England. The higher death rate in India did not include those who could not be cured in India and died on the way back to England. In England, infant and general mortality began to rise again after 1815, associated particularly with the slums in industrial towns. The spur for more active public health measures was the cholera pandemic which reached England in 1831. Opinion as to the cause was divided between insanitary conditions and contagion. Cleaning-up and quarantine were both recommended. But it was soon shown that the latter was ineffective, and that there was a clear association with poor conditions such as a contaminated water supply. All the western nations began programmes of sanitary reform.

The state of public health in India in 1826 was summarized in a paper presented to the Medical and Physical Society of Calcutta. The speaker said that the civilian administrators were as ignorant as the military about the way to prevent epidemics, and the doctors were kept busy treating 'calamities which might be often averted'. Simple measures were all that was needed to prevent

> the premature extinction of many vigorous Europeans, after being brought over half the circumference of the earth, to defend a country which becomes their grave.[8]

The majority of diseases were due to the miasma of decaying vegetable and animal material, accelerated by the excessive heat, which itself reduced resistance to disease. This miasma was primarily the cause of severe fevers, but, by absorption into the body through the skin and the lungs, it affected the liver and the guts, 'which are the seat of the principal diseases of India'. There was general agreement on the benefits of pure air, but the siting of British stations was often determined by military criteria: near water for easy transport of supplies, and surrounded by well-wooded country for defence. As the number of inhabitants increased, tanks were dug, fields were irrigated, and human and vegetable rubbish accumulated – disease was inevitable. The opening up of canals, 'as much from motives of benevolence as to increase the revenue', with consequent overflowing or deliberate breaking down of the banks, was another potent source of disease. All rivers were heavily contaminated, not only with human and animal bodies but serving 'as the common sewers of the wide regions which they traverse'. The ideal situation for a settlement would be on sandy soil on tableland where water could not stagnate nor trees grow near it. But wherever Europeans settled they determined to make gardens – digging ditches, planting trees, and fertilizing the land, so that 'fevers and cauliflowers may now be had in their seasons'. The severe heat was itself a direct cause of many disorders, but there were sensible precautions, such as abandoning thick European clothing, particularly by the soldiers. It was noticeable that, when off duty, soldiers tended to wear 'loose trousers, with a shirt over them descending to the knees'. The dryness of the hot winds could be counteracted by wetted tatties around the house. But when there was no wind these screens became useless. The punka, in crowded places, simply transferred respiratory excretions from one individual to another. The speaker himself had devised a 'Thermantidote' – a machine which emitted a stream of air cooled by passing through wetted and perfumed tatties, the motor power being provided by the servants.

Determined efforts could bring about general improvement. The situation at Howrah was described by one medical officer when he arrived in 1827:

> the whole place was very unhealthy, with stagnant tanks and undrained marshes; the roads were simply mud, and the people lived in hovels on a very frugal rice diet. By 1835 this had all been changed by the actions of the residents, with the help of the magistrate. The tanks had been filled, the marshes drained, and there were puckah [macadamized] roads and streets. By public subscription a native hospital and dispensary had been built for the relief of the poor.

Regular accounts of the pattern of disease in different parts of the country were now coming in from the medical officers. In 1823 a report on the villages in one of the Districts in Gujerat showed that fevers affected 1/6 men and 1/20 women, all with massive enlargement of the spleen; more than a thousand cases had been treated successfully with bark. Bleeding was necessary in some cases, but this was 'scarcely ever resorted to by the village natives in their rude practice'. Other cases responded to mercury, but, if pushed to salivation, this was harmful. Rheumatism was common, particularly in women. Eye diseases were 'innumerable'; the local clumsy operation for cataract sometimes succeeded, but sometimes destroyed the eye. Stone (bladder) was not uncommon, and was treated by the itinerant lithotomist. Liver diseases were not as frequent as in Europeans. In Indian troops, disorders of the spleen were ten times commoner than of the liver.

Chest diseases were rare, and acute pneumonia was unknown; consumption was one twentieth of that expected in a similar number of British inhabitants. Smallpox epidemics occurred every three years. Two-thirds of the susceptible were attacked, and half of them died; one-sixth of the rest were left unfit with 'eyesight affected, damaged joints, ulcers, or mental fatuity'. Vaccination had been introduced in 1812, and seven thousand had been vaccinated. Five years later none of them had been attacked. The medical officer urged that there should be a general plan for vaccination every 4-5 years. It would have to be at Government expense – 'the people are far too poor.'

Sporadic cases of scurvy had been noted in the jails and in villages among the poor and ill-fed, particularly in the cold season and after failure of the crops; when grain was scarce and expensive the dealers adulterated their stocks. Scurvy was now being increasingly recognized in Indian troops. Outbreaks were reported from regiments in various parts of India. Hindus (rice-eaters) were the first to suffer – they had little enough to spend on food from their meagre pay. Muslims, who were allowed meat, were protected, until rising prices cut off their supplies. Even when the diet was known to be at fault, religious scruples often prevented any change. The disease started with pain and swelling of the limbs, with dark patches on the skin and 'degeneration of the gums'. Mental depression was sometimes so great that it was difficult to persuade the men to accept sick-leave and go home, which was the best treatment – once at home they all survived. In those who had no means of support when away from the regiment the deaths were as numerous as the cures. On campaign British and Indian troops were equally affected. In the First Burma War and the storming of Rangoon (1824) the diet of the British consisted of putrid salt meat, biscuit 'animated with insects' and rum, but they were given priority for the supply of comforts for the sick, and they recovered more quickly. Hindus could not be persuaded to alter their diet of rice and dal (split peas) and there was a high mortality, increased when complicated by dysentery. Because a 'scorbutic taint' was so common, surgeons were warned of the danger of operations and the use of powerful drugs such as mercury.

'Burning of the feet' was a common disorder in Indians and was thought at first to be related to scurvy. It caused a good deal of disability and it was difficult to treat. The connection with scurvy was ruled out, and a 'native unguent' sometimes helped, but the aetiology remained unknown.

There were now detailed studies of the effect of climate on disease, with temperature records throughout the year related to morbidity in Europeans, including women and children. There was debate about the merits of cold bathing. Surgeons with West Indian experience advised against it, but in India it was regarded as the best preservative of health, for both Europeans and natives, young and old. Poor Indians used the Ganges but there was always the danger of alligators. Europeans and the higher classes stayed at home and had pots of cold water poured over them. It was important to sleep cool. There were many occasions when it was perfectly safe in the open air. Everyone should be in bed by ten, and up with the dawn. Mosquito curtains were essential to prevent being kept awake by the buzzing and the biting – 'on a close sultry day, after spending a restless night, tormented by mosquitoes, a person's blood ferments with heat.' A certain amount of exercise was necessary to preserve health, but it was one of the luxuries of a northern climate that had to be largely given up. 'Gestation' (being carried) in a palankeen was good, and a swing could be used indoors in the wet. Gentle massage ('shampooing') was also good. When the sun was directly overhead, everybody retired to their rooms until the cool of the evening. New cadets were advised to take eight yards of flannel with them, but not to wear it until advised to do so in India; they would then find it of great benefit. Ladies were warned that all the joints of their pianos should be secured with brass; they should learn how to tune them and take spare strings.

Heat stroke – 'the apoplexy of the hot winds' – continued to cause a high mortality. At one station the surgeon noted that the start of the hot season was marked by sudden deaths among the natives, and then indiscriminately among the Europeans, of whom seventeen out of two hundred died. The old soldiers were particularly affected – one sergeant with thirty-seven years service died on walking from the hospital to the grog-shop, a distance of about one and a half miles.

The mainstays in the treatment of fevers were still purging, bleeding and quinine, but there were many relapses and complications involving the spleen and the liver. Hindus had strong religious objections to post-mortem examinations, and, when this was respected (as it was in earlier times), important information was lost, and much disease was the subject of uninformed speculation. But, as post-mortems became more common, meticulous observations were made, although these did not yet lead to major therapeutic advances.

Cooling a patient with a fever made him more comfortable, and ice was extensively used when available. The need for a constant supply was a spur to the ice trade (p. 143 f.n.8) and to processes for producing commercial supplies of artificial ice.[9] Bleeding in the cold stage (at the beginning of the rigor) was thought to relieve congestion of the internal organs. But it was dangerous if practised excessively, and this did not make it easy to decide what to do in recurrent attacks. If there was active congestion of the brain, a small stream of cold water to the head was helpful. The patient only needed a little food – a little sago with sherry was enough.

Blood letting still played an important part in the treatment of many diseases, but the general application of this was now being questioned, with reports of patients undergoing venesection feeling faint, and begging that it be stopped. But there was a long tradition of bleeding for fever in Bengal, and this was accepted by Indians. There was little difficulty in persuading them to be bled. Many of them were influenced by the

> old doctrines of humoral pathology, and they are very ready to expect a cure by removing some of the bad blood. The grounds of their belief are of minor importance, when they lead to useful practice.

When prisoners were treated in the jail, those who had seen the immediate relief to their colleagues by losing a few ounces of blood requested that they should be bled too.

The policy of vigorous blood-letting was not followed by all surgeons. It might prevent some of the late complications, but it was thought to be unnecessary in most of the fevers in India. The patient was already weakened by the disease, and 'of all depressing agents, blood-letting is without question the most powerful'. If depletion was needed, eight to ten leeches worked very well. Whatever the timing of bleeding in relation to the stages of the fever it was recognized that all recovery was due to quinine. The practice of giving quinine without waiting for remissions was introduced and this 'put an end to the custom of bleeding'.

Surgeons were now kept busy with the increasing numbers of Indian patients who were referred to the hospitals for major operations when their own practitioners could do nothing for them. Indian surgery was still very limited. Honigberger, in Lahore c. 1840 (p. 225), found that Muslim surgeons were mainly concerned with the administration of ointments and plasters for external healing. They also had

> some razors, lancets, and pincers for drawing teeth, and cupping-apparatus. Of operations with other instruments they had no conception. They did not even know how to bind an artery, and amputation was a process of which they had never heard. My operations for the extraction of the stone seemed to them a miracle; they soon, however, became proficient in the operations of tapping and vaccination, for both of which they had a strong inclination.

But cases of nasal reconstruction were occasionally seen by Europeans. Honigberger had charge of a patient who had had his nose, ears and hands cut off for assaulting one of the King's sentinels, and whose

> nose had been so well restored in the mountains that we were all surprised, and confessed it could not have been better done in Europe (p. 173).

There were regular reports of major operations by British surgeons: lithotomies, amputations and removal of tumours of the jaws, orbit and other parts of the body. But there was always the problem of persuading the patients to submit to surgery – 'the timidity of Asiatics is often an impossible obstacle to the use of the knife.' Even with extensive experience of treating Indians, medical officers sometimes found it difficult to get details of their symptoms because of the nuances of the language, however well it was known. The term 'toop' [fever] was often used for a wide variety of symptoms.

> Moreover, the natives of this country, like other enslaved nations, are cunning and crafty in the extreme. Have they observed, that their medical attendant is fond of bleeding, leeching, or blistering, it is in vain that he will inquire, if they suffer from pain, they will deny it.

The open operation of lithotomy for stone (p. 170) was so much dreaded that patients of all nationalities delayed seeking advice. With the introduction of the instruments for lithotrity (crushing the stone inside the bladder) from France in the 1830s, Europeans were prepared to submit themselves to this new 'closed' operation, and therefore reported for treatment at an earlier stage. It was formerly believed that stone in the bladder was rare in Europeans and Asians in India, based on the dictum that

> it is a law of nature, that the more an organ, or system of organs, is called into action, the more it is liable to disease, which is but a derangement of its action.

In the tropics there was an intimate relation between the skin and the urinary system. With the increased action of the skin, there was a proportional decrease in the action of the urinary system, and this, it was thought, would reduce the formation of stones.[10] Based on this, surgeons did not at first bring lithotomy instruments with them from Europe. But now it was clear that stone was a common disease in India. The first lithotomy was carried out in 1826 at the Native Hospital in Benares. The surgeon thought, at the time, that Indian practitioners did not know of any operation to cure the condition. Then surgeons in other parts of India started doing the operation on both Indians and Europeans. In 1836 a series of fifty-two cases of lithotomy in Indians with seven deaths was reported to the Medical Society of Calcutta.

In 1798 the Superintendent at the Native Hospital in Calcutta reported two successful operations for cataract – the first by a British surgeon in India. The number of operations, by various surgeons, then rapidly increased, using European techniques. The classical Indian operation (p. 171) was condemned for the many disasters after 'the delay occasioned during the performance of incantations', so that 'they blind more patients than they cure'. A separate eye ward was opened, and then the Native Eye Hospital in Calcutta in 1816. Surgeons with special training were sent out by the Company to set up hospitals in other centres. In 1835 the first professor of ophthalmology was appointed at Calcutta Medical College.

A number of Company surgeons became interested in mesmerism, having learned the technique from the Hindus. Mesmerism had been used in France for some major operations since 1829, and for the first time in London in 1838. James Esdaile, a Company surgeon from Perth, who had joined the Company in 1831, read these accounts in India in the 1840s while convalescing from a serious illness. He was also influenced by his knowledge of Hindu practice. In April 1845 he started operating under mesmerism and, within a year, had seventy successful cases, including amputations, cancer of the jaws, bladder stones, cataract, and removal of large scrotal tumours. A local committee was set up, which reported favourably. He was given ten beds at the Calcutta Native Hospital, which became known as the 'mesmeric hospital', although the professor of surgery expressed his reservations. There were no deaths as a direct result of the operations, but about five per cent from cholera, dysentery and tetanus.

Esdaile also applied mesmerism to painful conditions, such as sciatica, with relief and no harmful consequences. He had many successful operations for scrotal tumours due to elephantiasis (p. 100 f.n.16) weighing up to 100 lbs. Thomas Colledge, a Company surgeon in China and founder of the ophthalmic hospital in Macao (1827), had had a patient, Hoo Loo, with a scrotum 35 inches long and 44 inches in diameter weighing 56 lbs. Operation was prohibited by local laws, and, with permission from the Company, the patient was sent to London. The operation in 1830 was carried out at Guy's Hospital before an audience of nearly 700. The mass was skilfully excised, but the patient became shocked and could not be revived.

In 1847 the technique of inhalation anaesthesia by ether reached India, and was at once found to be more reliable than mesmerism. In 1849 the special hospital was closed, by which time Esdaile had carried out 260 major operations. He continued operating, but under ether anaesthesia, until he retired to Scotland in 1851.

Acupuncture was never part of classical Indian Medicine (p. 11). Ayurveda gave instructions for treating enlargement of the spleen (malarial) by inserting long heated nails, but this is a very different technique. As seen by British surgeons, the actual cautery was applied over the spleen and small incisions were made into which needles were inserted for half an inch. Then large nails were heated, applied to each incision and sometimes plunged into the substance of the spleen. The first known reference to acupuncture in a European language was by a Jesuit missionary to China in 1671. The first medical treatise (1683) was by Willem Ten Rhijne, a surgeon with the Dutch East India Company trading to Japan. He exchanged medical information with Japanese physicians practising traditional Chinese medicine which had been introduced into Japan in the middle of the sixth century. He described their techniques of acupuncture and moxibustion (the application of burning mugwort, *Artemesia vulgaris*). Acupuncture first appeared in India in 1830, when Company surgeon F. H. Brett introduced it for the treatment of rheumatic diseases. He wished to add his testimony to the many on record, for he had used the method on himself with great relief. He had learned the technique outside India.

As well as general hospitals for Indians the Company had set up dispensaries in the Presidency towns; they were cheaper and more popular than the hospitals. From the 1830s they spread outside the towns, mostly dealing with out-patients, but with some beds and some operations:

> The peaceful and civilising influence of the work done in the dispensaries and by regimental surgeons on the frontiers of India has been in political importance equivalent to the presence of some thousands of bayonets.

By the early 1840s there were seventeen dispensaries in Bengal, treating 100,000 patients a year. In the dispensaries as well as the hospitals male patients always far outnumbered female.

On requests by influential Indians for medical help, Medical Boards would be instructed by the Presidency Governments to send out a surgeon. When pregnancy was suspected in a nobleman's widow, Mr Surgeon Ogilvy was asked to visit her

> to clear the doubt by feeling her pulse, and if there is any other mode where the point can be ascertained without any Dishonour to the Family.

Ogilvy's opinion was that 'a diseased state of the Abdominal viscera has been mistaken for Uterine Gestation'.

James Burnes, the Residency Doctor at Bhooj in Cutch, was sent to Sind in 1827 to attend the Ameer[11] at his request, and to promote goodwill for the British. Private reports suggested that the disease was not serious, and it was suspected that this was a purely political move. Burnes was received with great ceremony. All the officials were mounted on camels, and 'sugar, sweetmeats and opium, were daily issued in great profusion'. He was impressed by the taste and cleanliness of the (Muslim) Court, compared to the 'mixture of gorgeousness and dirt to be seen at the courts of most Hindoo princes'. His boots had been taken off at the door, but he determined to keep his hat on. He was questioned on his age and medical studies; there was disappointment when he was found to be so young (he was twenty-six). The patient had been ill for five months, and two of his brothers had died of, or with, similar complaints. The local practitioners had given up. Burnes found that the disease was not dangerous, and that it could be relieved, if not perfectly cured. The family were delighted that no operation would be needed.

Burnes was compelled to abide by the rule 'which requires the physician to swallow one pill before he administers another', and he had to go shares with the Ameer to overcome his distrust at taking medicine from a stranger.

> As my complaisance could not bring me to inflict on myself the nauseous dose more than twice, an unfortunate attendant was selected as the subject of experiment, and underwent, without mercy or necessity, such a course of continued sweating and purgation, as must have left on his mind and body, any thing but a favourable impression of the European method of practising physic.

Later, as the highest compliment they could pay him, the Ameers dispensed with the rule. They regarded this as so important that they sent an envoy to inform the Governor of Bombay, 'as an extraordinary proof of their confidence and friendship for the British'. By diet, general treatment and simple dressings Burnes was able to cure the disease in ten days. He attributed his success to the removal of the irritating substances that had previously been applied. He was also successful in predicting the exact effect of a dose of quinine on the same patient:

> a remedy hitherto perfectly unknown in Sinde, and the effect of which, as it scarcely ever fails in stopping the intermittent fevers of natives, I could generally foretell with a degree of precision that astonished them.

He went on to cure a number of other noblemen, and he would have been able to do more, but the Ameers seized the phial, and locked it away for their own future use. They refused to release it, even when he himself was dangerously ill with a violent attack of fever. He stayed for two and a half months, overwhelmed with flattery and hospitality, and had difficulty getting away, worn out by treating all the people who flocked to him. The rulers had heard reports of the success of vaccination, and they asked Burnes to help them to establish this in Sind.

Company surgeons had been largely responsible for setting up and staffing the Native Medical Institution in Calcutta with teaching partly in the vernaculars (p. 179). The change of policy from 1835 meant that all education should be on western lines, with English as the official language. In 1833 Governor Lord William Bentinck had set up the Grant Committee (under John Grant, the Apothecary General) to make recommendations for the medical education of Indians. The Committee reported in October 1834, pointing out the defects of the Native Medical Institution: there was no proper standard for admission, the period of teaching was too short, and there was no instruction in human anatomy (the students were expected to dissect a sheep); the final examinations were also unsatisfactory. The Committee advised that the Institution and the medical classes at the Sanskrit College and the Madrassa should be abolished. A Medical College for Indians should be set up to teach only western medicine.

The Committee was at first divided on the question of language. Those who supported Sanskrit had been teaching in Sanskrit since 1824. Those who voted for English pointed out that it was difficult to translate technical terms into Sanskrit and that there were a very large number of other Indian languages, most of which were understood by only localized groups of people. Also, Muslims and Indian Christians would object to the exclusive use of Sanskrit. With the decision in 1835 that English was to be the official language of India, the Committee decided in favour of medical teaching in English.

The Medical College of Bengal (Calcutta Medical College) opened in 1835 with Surgeon J. M. Bramley as its first Principal. Pandit Madhusudan Gupta, who was widely respected for his liberal views and had trained in both systems at the Native Medical Institution and later taught there, was transferred to the new College. Most of the teachers were Company surgeons with expertise in special areas of medicine. On 20 February 1835 the first fifty students entered the College; their books were supplied by the Company.[12] Other medical schools were then set up on western lines. In Madras (1835) Indians with a knowledge of Ayurveda were recruited by the Company surgeons in charge, and trained to teach western medicine. In Bombay (1837) the school under the auspices of the Governor, Sir Robert Grant, developed into the Grant Medical College in 1845. During their training, students visited the General Hospitals, the Native Hospital, the Company's Dispensary, the dispensaries for the poor, and the Eye Infirmary. These medical schools were designed primarily to turn out medical officers of subordinate grade for the army, with secondment to civil stations as required. In 1839 the first four students graduated from Calcutta and were appointed Sub-Assistant Surgeons in country districts.

In Bengal, at this time, there was a general move towards the English way of life and literature. But there was still some opposition by high-caste Hindus to training in western medicine, with its reliance on a knowledge of anatomy gained by human dissection. A great step forward was taken when the first dissection by a Hindu was carried out. On 18 January 1836 Pandit Madhusudan Gupta, accompanied by Dr Goodeve, the professor of anatomy, went secretly to an outhouse where, in the presence of four students, he dissected a body that had been procured for a lecture. This was celebrated by a salvo of guns from the ramparts of Fort William. Madras was more conservative, and, at first, no respectable Hindu would enter the Medical School which recruited mainly from Anglo-Indians and the lower castes.

The Grant Committee, while deciding that medical teaching should be in English, did not forbid the teaching, in English, of the Indian systems. Bentinck, like Hastings before him, was interested in Ayurveda, and would have been prepared to see it develop alongside the British system. But Bramley, at the Bengal Medical College, discontinued all Ayurvedic classes. There were no objections to this by Indians, and it seems that Pt. Madhusudan Gupta was himself undecided, realizing that Ayurveda had become stagnant, and that no further progress would be made by changing its teaching into English.

A few vernacular medical schools remained, of which Hyderabad was the most successful. Hyderabad had had a hospital and teaching school since 1595. The nineteenth century medical school was the result of the successful treatment of the Nizam in 1845 by Dr William Maclean, the Residency Surgeon. The Nizam requested the Resident to open a medical school to teach 'native youths, through the medium of their own language, the science of Western Medicine', with Maclean as the first Superintendent. At first students were slow to come forward. Teaching was by lectures and examinations, a system at that time utterly unknown. 'After prodigious labour over eight years, Maclean had trained seventeen men as qualified to practice, and these all acquitted themselves creditably.' A new general hospital was established about twenty years later. Teaching continued in Urdu until 1884, when it was changed to English. In 1921, the Hyderabad Medical School was converted into a College by the Nizam, and renamed Osmania Medical College.

After 1858 these first Medical Schools (Calcutta, Madras and Bombay) were upgraded to Colleges. Other Colleges were founded, and a secondary tier of Medical Schools was set up (p. 216). They all turned out practitioners intended primarily for the army. Indian College graduates first entered the Bengal Medical Service in 1855. All the graduates at this time went either into

Government service or into private practice, and so were not doing anything to help the majority of the people by serving in rural areas. In Government service they were only of subordinate assistant rank at a lower rate of pay.

It was the same in other scientific fields – Indians were being trained, but were then kept in subordinate positions. British scientific work in India had been mainly concerned with the field sciences for their political, military, and commercial advantages. From the middle of the eighteenth century there were increasing trigonometrical, topographical, geological, and astronomical studies 'to ensure the military, administrative and economic control of the subcontinent'. Bengal had been surveyed in 1767-71 by James Rennell, and the Great Trigonometrical Survey of India was started in 1818, continuing under George Everest, the Surveyor General, from 1830.[13] These resulted in important increases in knowledge of science in general, but did little to introduce western science to Indians. Surveying, in particular, was restricted to the Company's servants. At first this was to prevent the knowledge falling into the hands of their military rivals, but, later, there was formal prohibition of the instruction of any Indian in any kind of surveying. When, later, Indians were recruited for the official surveys they were always in subordinate posts. The first Indian apprentice for the Geological Survey was appointed in 1873, but in the nineteenth century Indians did not rise above the rank of Sub-Assistant.

In 1855 the Educational Despatch of Charles Wood (Lord Halifax), President of the Board of Control, recommended that European knowledge, including science, should be diffused, and that there should be five residential universities. These were founded in 1857 in Calcutta, Bombay, Madras, Allahabad and Lahore. The Medical Colleges became the medical faculties of the new universities. But even after this general reform of the educational system, there was still relative neglect of the teaching of science to Indians, and a failure to appoint, as had been recommended, scientific teachers to the universities. Indians were restricted to subordinate positions, and they had very limited facilities for independent research.

Notes

1 It was said that an Englishman who stayed any length of time in India became either 'sultanized' (corrupted by despotic power) or 'brahmanized' (emasculated by submission). Lord Wellesley represented the former and Jonathan Duncan (p. 149) the latter.

2 *The History of British India*, 3 vols., London (1817), of which the opening sentence is: 'Rude nations seem to derive a peculiar gratification from pretensions to a remote antiquity.'

3 *The Education Minute*, 2 February 1835

4 K. C. Sarbadhikari (Principal, Medical College, Calcutta) writing in 1961.

5 Preparations containing multiple ingredients; in earlier times the term referred to antidotes to poisons.

6 Homoeopathy was introduced into India in 1838 (p. 225).

7 The majority of the Company's surgeons were trained in Scotland (p. 117).

8 In the First Burma War (1824-26) the mortality was 3.5 per cent killed in action and 45 per cent died of disease.

9 Commercial mechanical refrigeration was not available until the 1880s.

10 But the greater the concentration of urine the greater the likelihood of stones forming.

11 *Amir*, commander, chief (Ar.), applied particularly to the Princes of Sind.

12 The knowledge of English required for entry was the ability 'to read, write and enunciate with fluency and facility, to analyse a passage in Milton's 'Paradise Lost' or works of a similar classical standard and be acquainted with Arithmetic as far as the rules of proportion'.

13 The peak was named after him in 1852.

Chapter Thirteen
The end of Company rule

The Company was now the effective government of British India, controlling the administration, the revenue and the army, although still technically a trading company with its headquarters in London. Criticism of its management of Indian affairs was increasing in Britain, and the commercial monopoly was abolished by Act of Parliament in 1813. The main commercial activity became the very lucrative tea trade with China through Canton. In return, the Company exported opium from India. The huge profits from the opium and tea trades largely financed the Company's rising expenses in India. China tried to put a stop to the import of opium, and it was banned by the Emperor in 1796 but the Company continued to smuggle it in. Chinese resistance resulted in the Opium War of 1840-42 in which the Chinese were defeated, and Hong Kong was ceded to the British at the Treaty of Nanking in 1842. When the Company's trading monopoly was finally removed in 1833 there was no other organization that could take over the government. The Company was given a new Charter to continue in administrative control for a further twenty years.[1]

At home, by 1823, the Company had about 2,500 employees in London centred round the East India Docks. There were very efficient medical arrangements for them, with the Poplar Hospital for Accidents at the docks and twelve medical officers. There was accommodation for thirty-six pensioners, petty officers, seamen or their widows, and twelve better-class houses for commanders or mates and their widows. The Company headquarters, East India House in Leadenhall Street, built in 1762, contained a museum and a library, with a keeper and a librarian, and lecturers in Hindustani and the diseases of hot climates.

Travel to India had been speeded up, with steam vessels expected to reach Calcutta in two to three months. The voyage, 'passing twice through the tropics in the 14,000 miles from Spithead to the Ganges', gave the passengers time to acclimatize. There were no luxuries, especially towards the end of the voyage, and discipline was maintained – 'temperance was the rule'. There were strict precautions against fire. Passengers who wished to reward good service by the crew were advised that 'pig-tail' (chewing) tobacco made a better present than cut tobacco as smoking was forbidden. The voyages were now being completed without outbreaks of scurvy. Much of the credit for this was given to canned food, but most ships carried lemon juice as well. On shorter voyages, the Company's ships were very comfortable:

> a cow on board gave four gallons of milk a day; there were fresh rolls, and a large stock of fowls, sheep and hogs, which were very cheap in Bengal.

In India a forced journey of a hundred miles could be covered in fifteen hours in a palanquin, but large numbers of bearers were needed. The electric telegraph was started under Dr W. B. (later Sir William) O'Shaughnessy in 1849. By 1854, there was a line from Calcutta to Agra, with extra thick wires to withstand the jungle, 'but it had none of the friendly charm of letter-writing'.

India in the early nineteenth century had one-sixth of the world's population with only 10,000 British, described by Governor-General Dalhousie as 'a handful of scattered strangers'. Children had to be sent home at an early age, and families might remain separated for years. William Huggins, an indigo planter in Bengal, noted the intense feeling of isolation in the relatively small British communities. Earlier it had been possible, for those who survived, to stay on in India to make a fortune, and then go home. But now, although the senior Company servants lived in luxury 'like noblemen in England', many others who could not afford to go home 'cherish a longing for England which gnaws within them, like a worm, and disturbs their peace'. Many of the young writers were soon in debt, and the young officers lived 'in genteel poverty, anxiously longing for war to cause casualties and accelerate their promotion'.

Even those who could live in luxury, such as 'officers and other genteel classes of society', were constantly reminded of the hazards to their health, in spite of:

> the palankeen, the punka, the tatty, and the light, elegant, and cool vestments ... with the numerous retinue of domestics, anticipating every wish, and performing every office, that may save the exertion of their employers. The untravelled cynic may designate these luxuries by the contemptuous epithet of 'Asiatic effeminacy'; but the medical philosopher will be disposed to regard them as rational enjoyments, or rather as salutary precautions, rendered necessary by the great difference between a temperate and torrid zone.

Added to the health hazards was the realization that the disparity in numbers of Indians and British made survival unlikely if there was any major uprising.

Some of the British concealed their anxiety under a load of administrative duties; others relied on alcohol and opium.

Indian habits, previously freely adopted, were discarded. Smoking was common, and it might even be advisable at certain seasons and in places where there were dangerous exhalations. But it was now thought to be 'degrading to become a slave to the hookah' (p. 250), and there were suggestions that it should be banned from society. It was 'beyond endurance, to see a great, lusty hooka-burdaar, insinuate the pipe of his long smoke into the delicate hand of a European lady'. In some countries, e.g. Syria, the local inhabitants seemed hostile to European dress, and it was 'better to appear à la Turque as soon as possible after arrival'. But in India it was now 'the extremity of bad taste to appear in anything of Indian manufacture'. If India had once been seen as 'the land of wealth, mysticism and wisdom', the British now increasingly despised it. Some of the brightest flowers of India had little smell – 'India is a place where everything smells except the flowers.' The wealth was seen to be in the hands of a few autocratic rulers, and its culture, including medicine, was stagnant.

As well as the ill-effects of the sun, the continuing high incidence of disease was ascribed to alcohol. A typical Staff Surgeon's report stated:

> The complaints most prevalent among the soldiers have been hepatitis and dysentery; and in almost every instance, might be traced to dissipation, and exposure to the sun, while in an intoxicated state.

Station libraries were established for NCOs and men in an attempt to keep them off the liquor. The young cadet was advised to avoid spirits and malt; his pay and allowances would cover a pint of wine a day, which was quite sufficient. But belief in the value of alcohol in illness persisted, and in an influenza epidemic among Europeans they were advised 'to drink deep in rosy port'. Temperance was now not solely a matter of health and morals, for

> in a vast empire, held by the frail tenure of opinion, and especially where the current of religious prejudices, Brahmin as well as Muslem, ran strong against intoxication, it was soon found necessary, from imperious motives of policy, rather than of health, to discourage every tendency towards the acquisition of such dangerous habits. Hence the inebriate was justly considered as not merely culpable in destroying his own health, individually, but as deteriorating the European character in the eyes of those Natives, whom it was desirable at all times to impress with a deep sense of our superiority.

There was less and less contact with Indians, and educated Indians tended to keep to their own culture. Some Europeans might live in India for years without being able to distinguish the 'hindoo' from the 'moosulman'. An authoritative guide was available:[2]

> The Hindoos are all uncircumcised idolaters, of ancient footing in India; their garments fasten on the left, and their collars on the right. They mark their foreheads and other parts with pigment; they wear beads and bracelets, with beads round the neck and threads across the shoulder. They bury their dead or throw them in the gunga [Ganges]. The Muslims are deists and followers of mohummud, in India for the last nine centuries, and our predecessors in conquest. They have beards and are generally fiercer, more masculine and robust than the Hindu (except the rajpoot tribe). Their garments fasten on the right, and the collars on the left. They wear no ornaments but finger rings. They bury their dead.

The British had always felt more affinity with the Muslim aristocracy than with Hindus, but now this started to change as Hindus were regarded as

> peacable citizens and obedient subjects under any Government that treats them with common decency. Their meekness of spirit and tranquillity of habit have a right to be considered virtues of no light account, as it is in a great measure to them that we are indebted for the security of our empire.

The general opinion was that they could be employed in confidential situations, and the better-educated could be very useful – 'pay attention to their lucky and unlucky days, particularly if your business depends on their zeal.' But they should always be under the supervision of the British.

There was some concern for the many ways in which Hindus could be offended. This was often due to ignorance, and manuals were available to guide the newcomer, e.g. the beckoning sign appeared like 'be off'; the newcomer should learn to extend his right hand, palm downwards, flexing the fingers repeatedly. A nod of the head was less respectful than a courteous gesture with the right hand, and the salute of a Hindu should always be returned, but never with the left hand, 'for reasons that are inadmissable here'.[3]

But, while being urged to be tolerant of local customs, the newcomer was warned that Indians would try to take advantage of too liberal an attitude:

> the arrogance and contumely with which the Bramins in the Carnatic [east coast] are allowed to treat Europeans, is almost proverbial.

It was essential to 'safeguard one's national honour and private comfort'. The strain of the hot weather and overwork, and the increasing truculence of petty Indian officials, often led to abuse of Indians by Europeans. It was better to leave redress to the magistrates, remembering that 'in certain points of honour, they [Indians] are probably more tenacious than ourselves'. Newcomers were warned to be constantly on guard against deceit and pilfering by servants. To prevent the grooms stealing grain, it was only necessary for a European to touch it. No servant, even the lowest, would agree to any task that was outside the custom of his caste. Since they regarded all Europeans as impure, the lowest standards in the kitchen were permissible. This seemed to be the pattern in the cities, but in the interior, where servants were scarce, they were more often long-serving, with mutual attachment to their masters.

Among all the rising antipathy there were many conscientious and able civil servants determined to promote good relations in the large areas that they administered. To further this they made themselves fluent in the local language. Instruction in local languages was spreading rapidly, especially to convince Indians that the courts of justice were running fairly. Hindustani/Urdu[4] was the most widespread, and it could have become the common language of the people. It was taught to the Company's servants, and grammars and dictionaries were compiled. But Persian was always preferred by educated Indians. Urdu became more persianised and restricted to Muslims, and from 1835 English was the official language.

Proficiency in interpretership was the first step in gaining promotion for young officers. Medical officers in charge of training Indian doctors had to show that they were capable of reading vernacular treatises of medicine. No medical officer could be a Vaccinator or carry out any Residency medical duties until he had passed examinations in Hindustani and the local language. Interpreters were appointed in both European and Indian regiments to help particularly with courts martial; there was sometimes confusion between the verbs to 'beat' and to 'kill' – the distinction could save a life at a court martial. Officers were always required to learn the local language, if only to prevent their men being able to insult them with impunity.

Young officers were advised that, when faced with a line of sepoys, 'there is not one among them, except the very lowest, who does not consider himself of a higher caste than yourself'. If a sepoy was struck, he might well step out of the ranks and kill the striker. But, if treated fairly, 'they will follow you to the mouth of a cannon, or to the top of the best defended breach'. No attempt should ever be made to interfere with their religion. Orders should be given consistent with religious views, but there were wide variations in these, and local information was needed to decide between religion and chicanery. There were instructions to show Company and military officers how to deal with requests from soldiers for leave to attend a feast, when the officer

> cannot be certain that, in granting the application, he is doing justice to the service, or that in refusing it he would not infringe upon the religious feelings of his troops.

The number of Anglo-Indians (p. 130) was increasing, but they could no longer hold commissions or appointments. Many prided themselves on their British origins, and it was thought that, in an emergency, they would serve loyally. They might be formed into a corps to hold the balance between the European soldier and the sepoy, each of whom considered the other inferior.

The (officially recognized) relations of British men with Indian women had changed. In the advice to the newcomer in 1810, concubinage was accepted as normal (p. 153). In 1825 it was decreed that no permanent connection should be formed with an Indian woman, i.e. bringing her under the same roof or tent; 'you will from that instant be held cheap, and in a manner degraded in society.' But for some, 'the regulation of the passions might be impossible in hot voluptuous climes', or only possible for those of strongly religious and phlegmatic personalities. Others held that this was just an excuse for debauchery. The best remedy was mental exercise: arts, science, hobbies, 'even amidst the luxurious plains of British India, uncorrupted or defiled by their glaring impurities'. Best of all was to learn Hindustani, and develop a taste for oriental literature. If a man wished to get married he should wait until he got back to England; after ten years service he would be entitled to three years furlough.

But Indian mistresses continued as an essential part of military life. The liaisons were mostly temporary, ceasing when the regiment moved on.

> The European soldier ... has generally a domiciliated *chere amie*, who cooks, washes, and performs every menial drudgery for *massa*, in health, besides becoming an invaluable nurse when he is overtaken by sickness.

If a man had children by an Indian woman, his sons could not be admitted to the Company's service, and it was equally difficult to provide for daughters.

A man could stipulate that there were to be no children, and the women had a traditional recipe. Abortion was also widely practised – usually quite safely. But there were still many half-caste children, who were despised by both races. Indian women played a large part in teaching the men something about the country and its languages. Their displacement by the conventionally brought-up young Victorian ladies of the 'Fishing Fleet' (p. 79) increased the alienation of the men from India and its people.

Missionaries were an even more powerful divisive force, with their attempts to convert Indians to Christianity. Up to 1813 the Company – the 'godless corporation' – had appointed chaplains for its own service only, and had forbidden missionaries entry to its territories for fear that they would unsettle the people. But in the Danish and Dutch settlements missionaries had an important educational influence, setting up printing presses, and translating religious and other literature into Bengali – 'the founders of modern Bengali literature'. British administrators in the early nineteenth century were mainly Christian, but they managed to achieve a close working relation with Indians, both Hindu and Muslim. They would encourage Indian religious ceremonies if these would help medically, as in the campaign against smallpox (p. 176). The orientalists, stressing the antiquity and importance of Hindu culture, had argued that Christian missionary activity was unnecessary.

Now in England there was increasing pressure to reform the uncivilized customs of the Indians – 'their religious system is one grand abomination'. Powerful moves by Evangelicals and Utilitarians ensured that permission for missionaries to enter India was included in the Company Charter of 1813, to spread 'useful knowledge and religious and moral improvements'. Their views spread throughout India, where some officials believed that a large Christian population would be a support for British rule. At first it was thought that if Hindus were allowed to retain their caste structure they would 'embrace Christianity without reluctance and in considerable numbers'. Less attention was paid to Muslims, who referred to all Christians as 'god-eaters', and were resistant to conversion.

There was intense missionary activity, but conversion to Christianity only occurred among the lowest classes – the 'rice' Christians, who had received food while under instruction during a famine. Some of these recanted when it was over, and were accepted back into Hinduism. At an annual country fair c. 1828,

> may be seen one or two zealous missionaries expounding the Christion religion, surrounded by a number of clowns with open mouths, who do not understand one word that is said, and who are probably attracted merely by the hope of gain. One or two converted natives always accompany these well-meaning missionaries; but I fear they have assumed a name and a creed of which they are perfectly ignorant.

This evangelicalism, with other measures of westernization, was widely thought by Indians as an attempt to Christianize them all. Several ruling Indian families sent envoys to London to state their grievances. The continued denunciation of Indian religion roused fierce antagonism and raised the popularity of the emerging nationalist movement (p. 227).

There was little conflict between Hindus and Muslims. For Indian writers at this time the Hindu/Muslim question did not exist. There might be local squabbles over religious places and clashing festivals, but

> the professors of both religions have acquired a habit of looking on each other with an eye of indulgence unusual in other countries between those who maintain such opposite tenets.

Major riots did not occur until the twentieth century.

The increasing size of the Company's armies, predominantly Indian with a very small proportion of European troops, had often suggested to senior officers the possibility of a large-scale mutiny. The first mutiny of the Company's sepoys had occurred in May 1764. It was ruthlessly suppressed, and twenty-four of the mutineers were blown from the mouths of cannon. In 1806 there was a mutiny when the sepoys had been made to wear hats instead of turbans, and to parade without their traditional forehead marks. They were afraid that these 'foolish reforms' were the first steps in an attempt to convert them to Christianity. The high-caste Hindus forming the bulk of the Bengal infantry resented the lack of proper bathing facilities on campaign and the order to wear sheepskin jackets in the cold weather. Their religion forbade them to travel overseas, and in the First Burma War (1823-26) there was a mutiny when the authorities insisted that they should go by sea.

When the Sikhs were finally defeated in 1849, Dalhousie annexed the Punjab instead of leaving it to the trained civil servants. He introduced the 'Doctrine of Lapse', to take under direct Company rule any Hindu State when the ruler died without a direct heir. In 1856, under this policy, he occupied the State of Oudh, which had always provided a high proportion of the Company's most faithful sepoys. In 1856 he was succeeded by Canning who carried out further westernizing measures which caused widespread resentment. The Company's Charter was renewed in 1853, but its powers were further reduced. Indian troops thought that this meant that the British Government was taking control and would impose Christianity.

Rumours were circulating that food and ammunition were being contaminated with materials forbidden to both Hindu and Muslim by their religion, so that anyone in contact with these would lose caste and be forced to turn Christian. The sepoys were further antagonized by some of their British commanding officers who were religious fanatics. They saw this, combined with the missionary activity, as an attempt to overthrow the Indian religions, and Christianize them all. This came to a head in 1857 at the time of the old prediction that the Company Raj would last a hundred years. It was exactly a hundred years since the Battle of Plassey and Clive's conquest of Bengal (p.102).

The Indian Mutiny (known in India as the Sepoy Rebellion) started on 26 February 1857. It remained localized to Bengal, and large areas of India were unaffected. Twenty-eight Indian Medical Service officers, all from the Bengal Service, were killed (nine of them at Cawnpore), and ten died. Many of the soldiers were invalided home, and this was the spur for the foundation of the Medical School and Hospital at Netley for training army surgeons, with special study of the diseases of India and other tropical climates. The medical officers noted the impressive rate of recovery of cases of compound fracture of the femur following gunshot wounds, compared with those from European wars. They attributed this to the use, in India, of the dooly (p.141).

The Mutiny was largely under control by the middle of 1858, but it confirmed all the criticisms in Britain of the rule of the Company in India – 'an Empire ruled by stockholders'. The Company had become more a military power than a commercial, its army, the largest in the world, had mutinied, and it had run up huge debts. It was held to be wholly responsible for the disaster. In April 1858 Disraeli proposed the transfer of the power of the Company to the Crown. There was a strong counter-petition from the Company, and J.S. Mill urged that a Government Department was a poor exchange for the personal traditions of the Company. But after three India Bills power was handed over on 24 June 1858. Queen Victoria gave her assent to 'An Act for the Better Government of India', to take effect on 1 September, which was the last day of authority for the Court of Directors. Canning became the first Viceroy, and in 1877 Victoria was proclaimed Empress of India. Canning had seen the difficulty of settling the country, and tried for moderation, but he was greeted with uproar at home and in India – 'Clemency Canning'. Gradually the strength of Indian resistance to Christianization was recognized.

The remnants of the Company continued until 1 June 1874 when it was formally dissolved, and the remaining shareholders paid off. The Chairman had been reduced to a small office and one secretary. On 18 April 1873 *The Times* said:

> it accomplished a work such as in the whole history of the human race no other trading company ever attempted, and such as none surely is likely to attempt in the years to come.

Notes

1 'It is the strangest of all governments, but it is designed for the strangest of all empires.' (Macaulay, 1833).

2 *The General East India Guide and Vade Mecum* (Gilchrist 1825).

3 The left hand is used for unclean purposes, such as making love and cleansing after defaecation; only the right hand is used for eating.

4 Urdu ('the language of the camp'), a mixture of Hindi and Persian.

VI
MEDICINE IN INDIA AFTER 1858

Chapter Fourteen
The role of the Indian Medical Service

By 1877 three-fifths of the land and four-fifths (240 million) of the population of India were under British administration, with clear lines of responsibility between London and Calcutta. The opening of the Suez Canal in 1869 had brought a huge increase in trade and prosperity. Communications in India had been greatly speeded up by the expansion of the railways, the telegraph and the postal service. The three Establishments, Bengal, Madras and Bombay,[1] continued with their separate armies and medical services, although the medical officers already regarded themselves as part of an Indian Medical Service.

The Medical Services were under the control of Central Government, but they had great influence, and largely determined the policy on medical education (which followed European practice) and public health. Their clinical responsibilities were firstly the care of the military, secondly the health of European civilians, and thirdly the health of Indian civilians. From 1800-39 the mortality of British soldiers in India was 84/1000, falling in 1879-88 to 16/1000. For the surgeons, before 1838, more than half their careers were ended by death or illness, and only one-third were still in service at retirement. In the period 1839-60, half were still in service, and in 1865-85 two-thirds reached the age of 55-58 and retired.[2]

The three armies were combined as the Indian Army in 1895, and, in 1897, the medical services became the Indian Medical Service, and the doctors took on military titles. In 1946 Indians made up 40 per cent of the permanent officers in the Service and the majority of the large number of temporary officers.

From the middle of the nineteenth century the pattern of the Medical Service was changing from a primarily military service to a civilian service, as the intervals of peace grew longer. The military surgeon now found himself with time for research, except when there were wars or major epidemics. By contrast, the civil surgeon would have responsibility every day for the local hospital and dispensaries for Europeans and Indians, the jail (from 1868 he was given executive charge of the district jails, as well as his medical duties there), the health of the police, his official patients, and often a large private practice.

Joseph Fayrer arrived in India, aged twenty-six, in 1850. He was soon sent on active service in Burma. He so distinguished himself that the Governor-

General, Lord Dalhousie, appointed him Resident Surgeon at Lucknow. In addition to his medical duties as Superintendent of the hospital, School Medical Officer, doctor to the Geriatric Home, and a private practice, he was Superintendent of the Government Garden and Assistant Resident (political) to reorganize the Provincial postal services and to take responsibility for the horses, camels, elephants and wild animals formerly belonging to the deposed King of Oudh. In 1859 he was appointed Professor of Surgery in Calcutta.

But it remained the policy of the Service that all its members were liable for recall for miliary service at short notice. Private trading and other commercial activities, which had been very lucrative, particularly for civil surgeons, were banned for the military surgeons in 1824 and for the civil in 1841. The wide range of duties of the civil surgeons left them little time for research, and many felt that it was only to be expected that the military surgeons would be the ones to make advances in the knowledge of tropical diseases. Major Ronald Ross was a military surgeon when he established the essential factors in the transmission of malaria[3] in 1897 (p. 220).

The recruits to the Medical Services now held the diploma of the College of Surgeons (p. 189), and an increasing number of them had university degrees. In 1844 the Royal College of Surgeons of England instituted a Fellowship; of the 227 elected, 29 were from the Indian Services.

The Medical Services were responsible for establishing the European pattern of medical education of Indians, and they provided most of the teaching staff and all the Directors of research institutions. At first there was a two-tier educational system. Medical Colleges, which awarded degrees, had been set up in Calcutta, Bombay and Madras in 1835, and later in Lucknow, Lahore and Patna. The students were mostly intended for Government service in subordinate roles, but the best graduates were eligible for posts in the Indian Medical Service. Their qualifications were recognized by the General Medical Council, and, from 1892, they were able to practise in Britain. By 1937 there were eight colleges awarding degrees, with 3,167 men and 305 women students. In the second tier were the Medical Schools, with a shorter curriculum. They were cheaper to run, and open to lower classes of students. It was hoped that these students, being more familiar with village life, would be willing to practise in the neglected rural areas. Up to 1930, eighteen Schools were founded, of which two were for women (1923); by 1937 there were 4,750 students. Hindus always made up the majority of the students. Muslims only reached proportionate numbers in the 1920s and 30s with reservation of places.

There was always the problem of getting the newly qualified doctors to work in rural areas, and many College graduates went into private practice. By the 1860s private practice was becoming scarcer and less profitable, and graduates were urged to join the Indian Medical Service where the standards were reputed to be higher than in some of the London medical schools. There was increasing pressure to dismantle the two-tier system; Indian nationalists felt that it implied a second-class system. The Schools were all gradually phased out or up-graded to Colleges.[4]

In Europe the science of bacteriology was developing from the 1870s but diseases such as cholera,[5] typhoid and malaria had already come under partial control by sanitary reform, with improvements in housing, water supplies and hospitals enforced by a number of Public Health Acts. In India, in 1859, a Royal Commission on Sanitary Conditions of the Army was appointed to enquire into the causes of the poor health of the sepoys. In all the wars in India, including the Mutiny, more soldiers died from disease than were killed. It was thought that their poor health was typical of the health problems of the Indian people generally, although there was no detailed information about the civilians. The report, in 1863, showed that sanitary conditions everywhere were appalling. Increasing urbanization was leading to crowded unhealthy cities. The countryside round every bazaar was 'one immense privy'. Bombay had a fair water supply, but no drainage. Madras had neither water nor drainage. Calcutta was being drained, but had no clean water; the river from which all water supplies were drawn was full of corpses, including those from the hospitals, which washed backwards and forwards with the tides. But it was thought that a ban on this method of disposing of corpses would be seen as an attack on the Hindu religion.

The Sanitary Act was passed, and its recommendations came into effect in 1864. The main object was to protect the military stations by improving living conditions of Indians living near by, without concern for the rest of the population. The Town Improvement Act of 1865 brought a start to the collection and disposal of sewage. Sanitary Commissioners were appointed in the three Presidencies, but they were subordinate to the Indian Medical Service with its concern for the military, and were not able to do much to improve conditions in the villages. Gradually, training programmes were introduced, but, although the rules of hygiene were recognized and some individual (relatively junior) officers made great efforts, there was no effective agency in the villages, and funds were always limited. The Army Sanitation Commission in 1887 showed that 80 per cent of all deaths were due to preventable disease.

The water supply was tackled next. The Sanitary Commission had reported on the water supply of Peshawar:

> I do not see how matters could be worse except in a community which drew no distinction between its cesspools and water tanks, and used each indiscriminately for all purposes.

But the supply was often installed before adequate drainage had been established. The resulting stagnant pools were breeding grounds for mosquitoes. Construction of canals made some areas fertile and habitable, but increased the mortality from malaria.

At the International Sanitary Conference in Constantinople in 1866 India was accused of being the source of cholera, and that the Government had failed to control this. The authorities were still excusing their inaction by the old 'orientalist' view that they should not interfere with customs such as the massive pilgrimages, even though these were one of the main routes for the spread of cholera. Calcutta got its first good water supply in 1870. Other cities followed, so that by the 1890s the incidence of cholera was reduced.

The village people were repeatedly held to blame for their unhealthy customs, their apathy and resistance to change. But in 1904 Central Government was still urging that the people should not be worried by forcing measures of hygiene on them. The main concern was always with urban areas, separating the cantonment from the native city to protect Europeans. After 1900 slum improvements were started, but these were opposed by the landlords and by the municipal authorities as too expensive.

Infants were the group with the highest mortality, and the rate remained stationary for the greater part of the nineteenth century – higher for girls than boys, with the general neglect of girls and selective infanticide until the Infanticide Act of 1870. Women after giving birth were regarded as unclean, and were therefore neglected. Women in purdah were poorly educated, living a monotonous existence with no exercise, leading to anaemia and osteomalacia, They were allowed no male medical attention and they refused to go to hospital. Their only care was by Indian midwives (dais), who were repeatedly criticized for being ignorant, dirty and incapable of learning; there were scattered attempts to train them, but these were not co-ordinated. Central Government generally showed little concern for the high mortality and morbidity in women and children, whose care was left largely to individuals and missionaries. The first medical women in India were American missionaries in 1869. They brought the problems to light, and were able to treat women in purdah. It was recognized that the only way to improve the service was to train women doctors and women subordinates, and to open special hospitals and wards for women. Support from Government slowly increased, and in 1875 the first women were admitted for medical training. The first all-women medical school was the Lady Hardinge Medical College in Delhi in 1916. The wives of successive Viceroys were responsible for raising funds for maternal and child health. The first professor of midwifery had been appointed by the Company at the Calcutta Medical College in 1841. Successive professors of obstetrics and gynaecology carried an increasingly heavy load, and, by the 1920s, men like V. B. Green-Armitage IMS (professor

1923-33), as well as working on infant and maternal mortality, were carrying out pioneering major operations of a sort much less common in Europe.

Medical research only became organized towards the end of the nineteenth century. Previous work by individuals had included detailed topographical surveys of the different regions of India, covering the geography of the country, its climate and produce, and the social conditions of the people as well as their medical state. Textbooks were published covering all the diseases of India, with more specialized texts on, for example, medical jurisprudence and insanity in India. As well as medical research, important work by members of the Indian Medical Service was carried out in zoology (animals, birds, fish, insects), botany, geology, archaeology, and in Indian culture and languages, with the production of grammars and dictionaries.

The spur for organized medical research was the re-introduction of bubonic plague (p. 221). After the Plague Commission had been set up, science and research councils followed for other health problems such as malaria and nutrition. These were financed by the Indian Council of Medical Research (1912) which was the prototype for the Medical Research Council in England (1916). In 1921 the School of Tropical Medicine was founded in Calcutta with Sir Leonard Rogers IMS as Director; there was a Chair of Pharmacology for research on the chemistry and therapeutic value of indigenous drugs. In 1924 Rogers set up the British Empire Leprosy Relief Association for research and treatment (p. 221). In 1929 Nutrition Research Laboratories began to study diseases in different communities on different diets to asssess their relationship. In 1932 the All-India Institute of Hygiene and Public Health was founded with Rockefeller money for training and research. Like the medical schools, these institutions were directed and largely staffed by officers of the Indian Medical Service who, later, would see as their main function the training of Indians to take over.

Most of the major scientific research was being done by Europeans. The Trigonometrical Survey had been set up in 1818, and the major scientific departments followed throughout the nineteenth century: Geological (1851), Meteorology (1875), and Botanical (1890). Indians were recruited, but they were restricted in the amount of responsibility they could take. The change came with the Universities Act of 1904, when the universities were required to set up facilities for teaching and research in science. This research, which had been largely restricted to the official scientific services, now passed to the universities. Before this, independent scientific research had been started by Indians, with the establishment of the Indian Association for the Cultivation of Science in 1876 by Mahendra Lal Sircar, a graduate physician and practising homoeopathist (p. 226) who was hailed as the 'founder of scientific research in India'. By the end of the century major contributions had been made in, for example, mathematics (Asutosh Mukherji), physics (J. C. Bose and

C.V. Raman) and chemistry (P. C. Ray). The Indian Institute of Science was founded in 1909, and a number of scientific research institutes were set up, often with the support of wealthy Indians.

As well as general public health and sanitary measures, individual diseases were tackled with support by grants from Central Government. Malaria parasites had been demonstrated in blood by Alphonse Laveran, a French Army surgeon, in 1880, and in 1897 Ross conclusively proved the link with mosquitoes, and that the disease was transmitted by their bites. The aquatic larval stage was then attacked by draining and treating breeding places, many of which had been created in the course of irrigation schemes and road, rail and canal construction. But in spite of all measures the mortality remained high. British troops in malarial areas in WW I were heavily affected. In WW II, under the direction of Indian Medical Service officers from the Malaria Survey of India, preventive measures with anti-malarial drugs reduced the incidence to a fraction of that of WW I in troops campaigning over the same terrain at the same season.

Kala Azar (Black Fever, Leishmaniasis)[6] was thought to be a form of malaria, having been known for centuries as epidemics of fever, wiping out populations so that the areas reverted to jungle. The only treatment was to leave the affected area. In its cutaneous form it was known as Delhi Boil or *Aurangzeb* after the Emperor who died of it (p. 101). In 1915 Leonard Rogers showed the efficacy of tartar emetic (potassium antimony tartrate), and then, even better, organic preparations of antimony which would cure nearly all cases if started early, where previously the mortality was 90 per cent.

Rabies was incurable but it could often be prevented by a vaccine if this was given soon after the bite of the rabid dog, jackal etc. The first vaccine was prepared by Pasteur in 1884, and for a time Paris was the only place where this treatment was available. There was always a high risk of rabies in India, and the Pasteur Institute of India was opened in 1900. By 1927 c.30,000 cases a year were being treated. After modifications in India the final form of the vaccine was adopted for general use in other countries. After 1938 the mortality of patients vaccinated was 0.2 per cent.

Snake-bite was a continuing problem; in Bengal in 1868 there were 1,144 deaths. By the end of the eighteenth century Patrick Russell and other Company officers had distinguished between the relatively few poisonous snakes[7] and the very much larger number of harmless ones (p. 95). The first systematic study was by Joseph Fayrer, professor of surgery in Calcutta, in 1872. He investigated the remedies recommended by both Europeans and Indians, and found them all to be useless. From the early twentieth century antisera were developed. In India these were found to be highly species-specific. A polyvalent serum was raised in horses, combining the four most poisonous species, which was purified and concentrated for distribution throughout the country, with wall-charts for hospitals and dispensaries for easy identification.

Cholera was endemic in India in the delta of the Ganges. From 1817 it began to spread rapidly through India and then outside. In 1831 it reached Britain where early attempts at control were based on the experience of surgeons who had served with the Company and knew that the disease was not contagious. In India in 1817-18 there were 150,000 deaths in the Company's territories alone. In November it hit the army on the march, and the roads were strewn with the dead and dying.[8] Since cholera was thought to be airborne there were regular army manoeuvres to avoid it. If possible, the troops would march at right-angles to the prevailing wind. In 'cholera-dodging', an afflicted unit would march out of barracks to higher ground and camp there, moving on to a new camp each day until there were no more deaths. Along the main roads there were small cemeteries at about twelve-mile intervals – 'marching cemeteries' – where the casualties were buried at the night's camp. All remedies were useless in 'true' cholera (p. 89). Attempts to counteract the collapse in the final stages by extra fluids and external applications failed.[9] W. B. O'Shaughnessy (later Professor of Chemistry at the Medical College, Calcutta) suggested intravenous saline, but, although this brought some temporary improvement, all the patients died, and the method was abandoned. In a cholera epidemic in Europe in 1883, Koch went out from Germany to India, where he identified the causative organism. The first sucessful treatment was by Leonard Rogers in the early twentieth century, using a modified intravenous infusion of saline made alkaline with sodium bicarbonate.[10] When this was given early, the great majority recovered. The most important public health measure was to identify areas where the disease was endemic, i.e, lower Bengal and the Yangtse Valley, and prevent spread from there by quarantine and sanitary measures.

Plague was re-introduced from China via Bombay in 1896 after the country had been free for over a century. In the next twenty years more than 10 million people died. The disease was spread by the improved methods of transport and by the urban poor who fled to the country. In 1899 the Plague Research Laboratory was set up in Bombay, with W. M. Haffkine as director. Earlier suggestions were confirmed that the disease was transferred from rat to rat by infected fleas, and then to man when the rat died. In 1926, the Laboratory became the Haffkine Institute with W. M. Bannerman[11] as Superintendent. The vaccine that was produced gave four-fold protection against attack, and six-fold against death in a vaccinated population.

The Leprosy Survey in 1877 showed an incidence of 54 per 100,000. In areas where it was prevalent, as in Colombo in 1806, the streets might be swarming with beggars covered with white blotches – 'one limb white, and the other the natural black'. The ancient Indian remedy, chaulmoogra oil, was introduced into Europe in 1854, but it was so nauseating that patients refused to take effective quantities. Later, hydnocarpus oil, another traditional remedy, introduced by Leonard Rogers, was more effective and less irritating. Rogers found that preparations of fatty acids derived from the two oils injected subcutaneously were the best, and these remained in use until the introduction of the sulphone drugs in 1942.

The treatment of stone in the bladder was advanced by (later Sir) Peter Freyer who served for 22 years in India. The 'closed' operation (p. 195) crushed the stone but left the bits in the bladder. Lithalopaxy, introduced from America, used an apparatus that removed all the debris. Freyer, from 1882 in Benares, treated over 600 cases by this method with a mortality of 1.8 per cent. After retirement to England in 1897 he devised the operation for enlarged prostate which was widely adopted and bears his name.[12]

From the 1860s the cataract operation was becoming standardized, and a widespread service developed. By 1928 Henry Smith at Jullundur in Punjab had treated 50,000 patients. His modified technique was practised all over India, and was copied by surgeons from other countries who came to study under 'Jullundur' Smith.

The Company's medical services, continuing as the Indian Medical Service, established western/modern medicine in India. The Indian Medical Service largely determined medical policy until it was disbanded at Independence. This policy has its critics as well as its supporters. The medical education of Indians was started early and spread widely, so that they made up the greater part of the country's medical services, laying the framework for medicine after Independence. But the teaching was on European lines, concentrating on individual diseases rather than general problems – 'one-to-one' medicine rather than public health. The main clinical concern was the health of the military, and then of European civilians; next came urban Indians, and finally, and sometimes only in major epidemics, the villagers. But the introduction of vaccination was 'one of the greatest victories medicine ever gained over disease'.

The British were criticized for maintaining large armies which took up so much of the available health-care, and the Service was criticized for its relative neglect of the public health and sanitary measures that would have improved conditions for the rural poor. Sanitary work did not rate highly in the assessment for promotion in the Service, and so perhaps was not a priority for its young officers. Under Central Government, sanitary officers were appointed, and plans were drawn up, but these were often frustrated by lack of funds. When power was devolved to the Provinces in the 1920s (p.227) local governments with nationalist policies made attempts to improve sanitation, but these again were ineffective from lack of funds. With the growth of urbanization the towns became even more crowded and unhealthy, while the villages became more impoverished. British civil servants were unwilling to serve in the smaller district towns if there were only Indian doctors to look after their families.

The development of the transport system was primarily for military reasons, but the railways, roads and canals improved living standards and allowed greater mobility to the people. Some areas were made habitable, but poor drainage systems at first increased the incidence of malaria. Improved transport and timely planning allowed rapid relief of famine, but in an epidemic, such as plague, it meant that fleeing urban populations spread the disease more widely. After the great Bengal famine in 1943 efficient transport meant that deaths from starvation were soon curtailed, but there was an increased mortality from intercurrent diseases over the next few years.

At all times it was recognized that there were problems in trying to change the way of life of the majority of Indians, whose culture encouraged passive acceptance of hardship. Caste rules had taught them their duties, not their rights, and by tradition they expected little from public services. They followed customs that were often unhealthy, and they were resistant or even hostile to change.

Notes

1 Referring to each other as 'Qui-his' (Bengal), 'Mulls' (Madras), or 'Ducks' (Bombay): *'Koi hai'*, calling servants, 'is anyone there?' (Bengali); 'mulligatawny', pepper water (Tamil); 'Bombay Duck', small dried fish.

2 Figures compiled by D. G. Crawford, Lt. Col. IMS, who was born in the year of the Mutiny, served in the Bengal Medical Service, finally as Civil Surgeon, Hughli, and survived to write the history of the Indian Medical Service up to 1913.

3 For which he was awarded a Nobel Prize, the first in Britain.

4 At Independence it was decided that there should be only one type of 'modern' medical education.

5 In 1854 John Snow showed that the 'poison' of cholera was water-borne.

6 Due to a parasite carried by the Sand Fly.

7 One of the commonest of these was given the name 'Russell's Viper'.

8 *Cholera morbus* – known to the troops as 'Corporal Forbes'.

9 It was not recognized that fluid replacement was only effective when given intravenously.

10 To those who still doubted the water-borne transmission of cholera, Rogers would say, 'You can eat cholera, you can drink cholera, you cannot catch cholera.'

11 His wife, Helen, wrote *Little Black Sambo*.

12 For its success in relieving urinary obstruction it is sometimes known as the 'pee freer' operation.

Chapter Fifteen
The revival of Indian Medicine

With no official British support since 1835 the social position of practitioners of Indian Medicine had declined. Indian rulers who had supported the classical systems were losing their authority with the spread of 'westernization', and patients were finding that modern medicine was more effective. But there were still many Indian practitioners, Hindu and Muslim, and they greatly outnumbered the 'modern' registered practitioners, A few vernacular medical schools remained, such as Hyderabad (Muslim) (p. 200) and Lahore (teaching both Ayurveda and Unani), with some courses adding basic science teaching.

In 1907 the All-India Ayurveda Mahasammalan, a national representative council, was formed. This was joined by the prominent Muslim, Hakim Ajmal Khan, who founded the Unani College in Delhi, which was opened by the Viceroy in 1916. But other requests for support were turned down. In the inter-war years, new indigenous colleges were founded with good financial support by Indians, and trained practitioners were first registered, on a separate register, in Bombay in 1938. There was opposition from 'modern' practitioners, particularly to homoeopathy which was being spread in India by homoeopathists from Europe, and was becoming increasingly popular.

Homoeopathy,[1] founded in Europe by Samuel Hahnemann towards the end of the eighteenth century, was brought to India by John Martin Honigberger in 1838. Honigberger, from Transylvania (E. Hungary), first reached India in 1829, becoming one of the personal physicians to Ranjit Singh, the Sikh ruler in Lahore. He had a very lucrative practice, and, as was the custom, was given charge of an industrial concern – in his case, the gunpowder factory. In spite of this he was 'affected with nostalgy', but he had considerable difficulty in getting Ranjit's permission to leave. Back in Europe in 1834 he heard that a new method of curing disease had been discovered, and he went to study with Hahnemann, becoming a fervent homoeopathist. From 1836-8 he was in practice in Constantinople, where he received a message from Ranjit asking him to come back. He remained in Lahore until Ranjit's death in 1849.

Honigberger wrote scornfully of the superstitious practices of the local physicians:

> sometimes I could not forbear laughing, when at consultations with the hakims; but I thought that when among wolves one must howl also.

But he urged the study and use of local plants, and he tried out some of the local remedies and found them to be effective. He was in charge of the local hospital, but the hakim was set up in practice on the other side of the building, and patients would often visit them both, and take both their medicines. Ranjit himself also had Hindu practitioners on his staff, so that he was accustomed to take three medicines for every complaint; the hakim's favourite prescription included powdered pearl and other precious stones (p.244). Honigberger went to great trouble to convince his patients that his own remedies would at least do no harm:

> [alloeopathia] rushes into the field, armed with enormous pills, and bottles of all sizes, containing the most powerful mixtures, striking at the foe with wild and deadly force; [homoeopathia] with less martial display, attacks the enemy in a manner which seems the quintessence of feebleness and inertia – a small case, containing pygmean flasks, filled with lilliputian pills which the least breeze would scatter to the winds, and a few minute drops, are all the direful weapons.

He gave most of his medicines in the dry state, as Sikhs and Hindus would not take any medicine prepared with liquids by European hands. The hospital in Lahore employed Hindu attendants for this purpose, and provided water from the Ganges.

Homoeopathy was at first regarded in India as quackery and beneath the dignity of qualified practitioners, but it gradually spread, particularly in Bengal where Homoeopathic Colleges were set up in the late nineteenth century. One of the pioneers was Mahendra Lal Sircar (1833-1904) who had qualified in medicine in Calcutta. Starting his practice in 'modern' medicine, he was impressed by the benefits of homoeopathic remedies, and became converted. He tried against great opposition to convince other practitioners, but he was boycotted at the annual meeting of the Bengal branch of the British Medical Association of which he was a vice-president. He was ostracized and lost his practice. But his efforts resulted in the spread of homoeopathy, both by locally-trained students whom he inspired, and by practitioners coming out from Europe. Since there was no Homoeopathic College in India at that time, some students went to America to qualify, and then returned to practise in India. In spite of the opposition to his advocacy of homoeopathy, Sircar was widely known and respected for his promotion of scientific reasearch (p. 219). He died in 1904, refusing to the last the catheterization that might have saved him, because it was against his homoeopathic principles.

From the early 1800s some British administrators had foreseen a time when India would be self-governing. The education programmes set up by the Company in this 'orientalist' period (p. 152), with their emphasis on equality and liberal ideas, influenced young Indians, particularly in Bengal, towards what would become a rising nationalist movement carrying Indian Medicine with it. The number of Indians entering Government posts steadily increased.[2] In 1861 the first Indians were appointed to the Viceroy's Advisory Council and to the High Court Bench. The Indian National Congress, founded in 1885, was a powerful force in the nationalist movement.

The Morley-Minto reforms in the 1919 Government of India Act largely transferred power, including health policy, to the Provincial Governments which became responsible for medical education, although Central Government remained responsible for standards. This gave increased power to Indian ministers, many of whom, with other nationalists, supported Indian Medicine which had the advantages of cheaper education and lower running costs. The number of students applying to read western medicine was increasing; those who were not accepted often enrolled in alternative colleges, mainly the Homoeopathic Colleges. This was beginning to set the pattern for medicine in the post-Independence constitution.

Between 1912-17 a number of Medical Acts set up Medical Councils in the various Provinces, and laid down qualifications for registration of medical practitioners, which excluded traditional physicians and made it illegal for a registered practitioner to be associated with Indian Medicine. The first 'Committee on Indigenous Systems of Medicine' was set up in Madras, reporting in 1923. It recommended that, as Indian Medicine was the best way of reaching most of the people, it should be developed to include recent advances, with proper training schemes and facilities for research. No action was taken on this. In the 1930s and 40s a number of other committees were set up to study and encourage Indian Medicine.

In Central Government some wanted to exclude Indian Medicine completely, feeling that it was based on a faulty hypothesis, and that this would never change. As an example, the emphasis on prognosis in Ayurveda was quoted, with its teaching that when a disease was recognized as incurable it should not be treated (p. 8); this was regarded as unethical. Others supported medical schools that integrated Indian and western medicine, recognizing that their graduates 'for many years to come, will constitute the medical attendants of by far the largest portion of the Indian community'. But the Medical Registration Acts meant that doctors from integrated schools would face de-registration.

Both views were represented in the Indian National Congress, with the 'modernisers' and western-style doctors supporting western medicine. Resolutions supporting Indian Medicine were passed, but through the 1920s no definite commitment to either was reached. In 1928 the Indian Medical Association was founded, calling for joint registration, but recognition of Indian medical degrees by the General Medical Council in London demanded a clear distinction. This, with the financial restrictions and opposition by the Indian Medical Service, meant that indigenous colleges got little support,

The rise of Indian Medicine was handicapped through the 1930s by disputes between the supporters of the different classical systems. Each group insisted on its own theory of practice and its own training-plan. They were also divided by the debate between those who favoured an integrated system, and those who insisted on pure indigenous medicine – a debate that continued after Independence. The vaids and hakims would not act together, although they were united in their opposition to the homoeopathists and the folk-practitioners.

The definitive committee on the health services, but excluding Indian Medicine, was the Bhore Committee,[3] set up 1944, reporting in 1946. The Committee recorded the health conditions in 1944, noting the high mortality, particularly infant and maternal, the short life-expectancy, and the high incidence of disease. Much of the disease was due to poor sanitation, lack of clean drinking water, poor nutrition, lack of health services, and poor health consciousness in the people, and was therefore largely preventable. All these factors were worse in the rural areas than in the towns. There was a shortage of all health workers, hospitals and dispensaries, and most of these were in the towns where 75 per cent of the doctors practised.

The Committee recommended a system of socialized medicine under the control of individual States. Health care should be for all, regardless of ability to pay, with particular attention to rural areas and emphasis on sanitation and prevention of disease. Training of doctors should be changed in all Medical Colleges to include social and preventive medicine.

A number of governmental committees had been set up through the 1930s to consider policy on Indian Medicine, but no decision had been taken. The Bhore Committee only dealt with western medicine. After widespread criticism, the Chopra[4] 'Committee on Indigenous Systems of Medicine' was set up, reporting in 1948. Chopra recommended that the indigenous systems should be integrated with western medicine, so that students of Indian Medicine were taught those aspects of western medicine that were not part of Indian Medicine, e.g. public health, surgery and ophthalmology.

This was the position when medical policy was debated after Independence.

Notes

1 After 1947 homoeopathy was one of the five officially supported systems of Indian Medicine.

2 By 1933 37 per cent of civil posts were held by Indians.

3 The Health Survey and Planning Committee under Sir Joseph Bhore.

4 Sir Ram Nath Chopra, professor of pharmacology and an authority on Indian drugs.

Chapter Sixteen
Independence

Independence was declared at midnight on 14 August 1947, with Jawaharlal Nehru as the first Prime Minister. The Indian Medical Service was disbanded, and control of the medical services handed over to State Governments. As the medical policy developed, six separate systems came to receive official support from Central Government and local State funds: modern medicine[1] and the five that make up Indian Medicine – Ayurveda (Hindu) including Siddha which is practised mainly in South India, Unani (Muslim), Homoeopathy, Naturopathy (the system favoured by Gandhi who was opposed to Ayurveda) and Yoga. Each system has its own practice and training scheme; they often have separate hospitals, or two systems may work on opposite sides of the same building. They all run a large number of dispensaries. All treatment is free.

Science was always strongly supported by Nehru, and the Council of Scientific and Industrial Research was set up. This led to a chain of national laboratories, and, later, atomic research and a space programme. From 1947-59 fifteen new universities and four higher institutions, with power to award degrees, were established, as against nineteen from 1857-1947.

With the country's limited finance, the health services had a relatively low priority, and the targets set by the Bhore Committee (p. 228) were over-optimistic. The objectives were water supply and sanitation, control of malaria, preventive care in rural areas, care of mothers and children, training and health education, self-sufficiency in drugs and equipment, and family planning and population control. In the budget for 1951-6 the share for health was 5.9 per cent. This was gradually reduced, reaching 2.1 per cent in 1974-9. The largest part of this (35 per cent) was for water supply and sanitation. Indian Medicine received 0.29 per cent, and family planning 0.5 per cent. All medical facilities, including hospital beds, were restricted by limited finance and the rapid growth of the population. The integration of the Princely States at Independence had increased the population by 93 million; the total by 1951 was 360 million and by 1961 439 million. One of the main recommendations of the Bhore Committee was that the people should be involved and educated in simple health precautions. Citizens' Committees, were set up in the villages, but they were poorly supported, particularly by the doctors, and had little effect.

The general mortality has been lowered, although infant and maternal mortality have always been proportionately higher. Life-expectancy has increased – in 1911 it was 23 years for men and women, and in 1961 45 for both. But by 1978 90 per cent of the villages still lacked water and basic sanitation; there was better provision in the towns, but then only 34 per cent. There are measures to control smallpox, cholera, plague and malaria (the incidence started to rise again after 1965), and effective famine relief. Tuberculosis has increased, with a high mortality, and has proved difficult to control.

There has always been the difficulty of getting trained doctors to practise in rural areas. If they go out to the villages there are few facilities for sophisticated medicine. It is all simple preventive medicine and not much else. Young doctors with families feel very isolated. They might fail to understand the village culture, and find it easy to blame the apathy of the people and their resistance to change. There is little opportunity for further training.

The western-style training, with its emphasis on person-to-person curative treatment of individual diseases (p. 222), turns out trained doctors rather than primary health carers. The 'westernized' doctor has little appreciation of the problems of the rural poor. Most of the graduates, modern and Indian, tend to remain in the cities, and some rural areas may still be served by the type of folk-medicine that has persisted since Vedic times.

> The departments of Social and Preventive Medicine attract the less successful or the unmotivated, while irrelevant and expensive super-specialisations are the goals of the best and the brightest.

In Ayurveda, Unani and modern medicine there is a statutory period of training of five years, with a compulsory six months internship at the end of it. For Homeopathy and Naturopathy the period is four years without the internship. During their training, modern students have no exposure to Indian Medicine, but the Indian training includes nine months of modern pathology, therapeutics, surgery, dental surgery, ophthalmology and public health. Since 1971 training and practice of Indian Medicine have been controlled by the Central Council of Indian Medicine.

In 1969 the Central Council for Research in Indian Medicine and Homoeopathy was set up with particular responsibility for the evaluation and standardization of traditional herbal drugs. These are collected directly from the forests by the teacher, who takes his students with him. The plants are not grown in special plots except for identification as they lose their power in an unnatural habitat. The Indian pharmacopoeias are being worked through with modern pharmacological techniques in the search for cheap, effective and relatively harmless indigenous drugs, in contrast to expensive modern drugs, which often have serious side-effects. It is claimed that among drugs in modern use which have been derived from the Indian pharmacopoeias are picrotoxin, emetine, strophanthin, serpasil and cocaine.

These research programmes are opposed by the traditionalists in Ayurveda who hold that their medicine came originally from the gods, and that nothing should be allowed to alter it. It is a fundamental principle that their remedies shall do no harm. They claim that they have learned, by experience over generations, the safety and therapeutic effects of a plant or part of a plant, either by itself or in combination with other plants. If these plants are broken down into their constituent alkaloids, the active extract might well have toxic effects which do not occur when the plant is intact. This accords with the Unani concept that 'certain corrective substances are all present in the crude drug which are removed during isolation of the active principle', but the Unani practitioners are generally more sympathetic to modern research than the Ayurvedic.

The more 'scientifically-minded' practitioners would like to see their treatment improved by any scientific method that would benefit their patients. Scientific validation would also increase the status of Indian Medicine in the eyes of modern physicians. There have been suggestions that the classical *dosas* (humours) can now be identified in modern biochemical terms, e.g. *kapha* as histamine. This dispute about research in Indian Medicine is an example of what has been described as 'the old Indian controversy' of Gandhi versus Nehru – nineteenth century conservatism versus the doctrine of 'take the best part of all systems'.

Indian Medicine deals more with chronic than acute disease. There is very little surgery, and no emergency or accident work. All acute conditions are referred directly to the general hospitals. Patients who are dissatisfied with either system are free to transfer from one to the other.

Diagnosis is made mostly on symptoms, but with some modern investigations, e.g. biochemical analysis and X-rays. Treatment is directed to the relief of symptoms, and is based on traditional remedies, mostly herbal with some mineral and metallic ingredients; all Unani preparations are made up with honey or sugar. Modern drugs are increasingly used, particularly antibiotics. Medication is combined with traditional physical methods, e.g. massage and oil inunctions. Mental factors in disease have always been a particular concern of Unani medicine.

Yoga is studied by measuring biochemical levels before and after treatment. Joint clinics with modern physicians assess its value in conditions with a 'stress' factor such as anxiety states. There has been success with asthma, and relief in, for example, cases of hypertension and thyrotoxicosis with 'stress' overlay.

In the Naturopathy hospitals the treatment is basically the same for all conditions – elimination of toxins by a raw vegetable diet, fluids, enemas, mud-packs, hot and cold baths, exercise and yoga, together with prayers and meditation. It is a preventive regime which the patient is expected to follow at home. The common causes of admission are obesity, 'servicing' (elimination of toxins), constipation, diabetes and hypertension. Some patients are referred from the general hospitals, usually to lose weight in hypertension or pre-operatively. There may be a modern-trained doctor on the staff or on call. Any patient who develops a complication, e.g. in diabetes, is transferred at once to the general hospital. When the crisis is over the patient returns.

There is less official transfer the other way. Modern-trained Indian practitioners are generally opposed to Indian Medicine. But for a disease for which there is no known treatment the recommended traditional drug may be given. If modern treatment has failed, patients will occasionally be referred.[2]

Indian Medicine borrows a good deal from modern medicine, not only in training and research, but in practice. Most hospitals have modern methods of diagnosis – X-ray equipment and biochemical laboratories. The Meditation Hall (for yoga) may be next door to the Whole Body Counter. Susruta's classical treatment with medicated threads for fistula (p. 10) is now regularly used but is under X-ray control with radio-opaque material.

Ayurveda and Unani have many features in common which were already established by the sixteenth century (p. 11). The vaid will tell you that Unani has borrowed so much from the Hindus that the only way now to tell the difference is by the amount of sugar or honey that the hakim adds to his preparations to make them more palatable – Unani medicines are notoriously sweet. The hakim will retort that the only thing the Hindus ever contributed was a superior supply of aphrodisiacs, from their greater experience of the needs of their patients.

Both systems are now required to incorporate parts of modern practice into their training programmes. Only Siddha medicine is consistent in keeping to the traditional methods of diagnosis and treatment. They all stress that their traditional drugs do no harm, and they contrast this with the dangerous side-effects of many modern drugs.

As well as the training schools in Indian Medicine, there is the long and continuing family tradition of folk-medicine, handing down the knowledge and skills from father to son, as it has done for generations. Like family medicine in all parts of the world, secrecy is an important part of the tradition. It is not unknown for a father to refuse to pass his knowledge on to his son, for fear that the son will take up modern medicine, and all power will be lost.

Notes

1 'Modern' is the term used in India today – or sometimes 'allopathic', to distinguish it from homoeopathy. Up to 1947 it was commonly called 'western' medicine.

2 Some years ago in Madras the author was told, by an orthopaedic surgeon, of a local family who know how to heal un-united fractures. Surgeons would send cases to them. The results are successful but the method remains secret.

EPILOGUE

Although much of the past activity of the British in India is seen by Indians as exploitative, they concede that the British conferred lasting benefits by the system of medicine that they introduced:

> the British laid the foundation for a principle neglected since Ashoka[1] that the health of the people is the responsibility of the State. This concept and the technology for fulfilling it was a British legacy to Independent India.[2]

This western/modern medicine was brought to India by the East India Company and continued and developed by the Indian Medical Service. It is based on the concept of disease as a separate entity more or less independent of the patient, his constitution and his way of life.

Flourishing alongside this are the traditional systems of Indian Medicine, based on the theory that disease is an abnormal state of the patient due to an internal imbalance – the 'humoral' doctrine that continued in Europe until the mid-seventeenth century.

Modern medicine aims to restore health by treating a disease. Indian Medicine aims to maintain health and prevent disease by a 'holistic' regime for the patient, his life-style – with particular emphasis on diet – and his environment. Disease is treated by correcting any imbalance.

The concept of disease as a separate entity was supported by the development of bacteriology in the late nineteenth century. But before this, and before powerful modern drugs, sanitary and public health measures brought about a general improvement in health. This showed that disease could be controlled by controlling the environment.

Today there is increasing emphasis on environment and life-style in the prevention of disease. The high incidence of a psychosomatic component in illness is now generally recognized, with the possibilities for improving the physical condition by relieving mental stress.

Patients have always been ready to move between different medical systems when these are available. Now many patients in the West are turning to alternative/complementary systems that have the 'holistic' approach that is the basis of traditional Indian Medicine.

Notes

1 Emperor Ashoka (279-236 BC) (p.12).

2 Srilatha Batliwala, 'The historical development of health services in India' (1978).

APPENDIX
Botany and drugs in India

The trading companies always encouraged the study of local plants and materials, mainly for their possible commercial value, but also for medicinal use. The classical Indian medical texts give lists of up to five hundred medicinal herbs and other substances. It was soon recognized that Indian physicians knew a great deal about the medicinal properties of their local plants, and that they also had special skills with metals and minerals, which was

> surprising, considering that fuel is very scarce, and that cow-dung cannot produce that degree of heat necessary for the fusion of metals.

The first European to make a systematic study of Indian flora, primarily for its medicinal value, was Garcia da Orta in the sixteenth century (p. 24). But little was known to western botanists until the publication in Holland in 1678 of the *Hortus Indicus Malabaricus*, the foundation of Indian botany, containing more than three hundred plants used in medicine. This had been compiled by Henrik van Rheede, the Dutch Governor of the Malabar Coast, with the help of local practitioners.

Botany was the first scientific study by the English Company's surgeons. Towards the end of the seventeenth century they started to collect local medicinal plants. The most assiduous collector in Madras was Dr Samuel Browne who was in the Company's service for seventeen years. He claimed to have collected every herb within a forty-mile radius. He noted 'the medical Vertues' of each specimen together with the local uses of the plants and the methods of preparing medicines from them, adding notes from his own experience. He listed a wide range of diseases: fevers, pox, rheumatism, worms, convulsions, gout, child-bed distemper etc., with numerous preparations for the cure of each. The collections of dried plants that he sent home were presented by the Company to the Royal Society in 1698 'for the benefit of the Publick'.[1] When any of these new drugs were found to be effective in England greater quantities were sent for from India:

> so that even the poorest sort of People may receive benefit

> by it at a more moderate price, and the Merchants receive advantage by trading in a new Commodity.

This and other studies by Company surgeons – particularly John Fryer in Bombay (p. 81) – established the properties of some of the commoner Indian herbs but there was still a large range unexplored. A detailed study at the hospital at Fort St. George between 1755-77 by Edward Ives and other surgeons discovered a number of remedies 'totally unknown to our brethren of the faculty in India'. Their properties were learned by consulting local practitioners and by clinical trials. There were 162 specimens, of which 80 had medicinal properties, most commonly for fevers (17), venereal disease (7) and flux (6). There were also remedies for bruises and wounds, worms, 'the itch', ringworm, snake- and scorpion-bite, colds, headache, cough, 'berbiers' (beriberi), consumption, swellings in the groin and dropsy, as well as details of purges, emetics, tonics and poultices.

In 1778 the Company appointed as Naturalist in Madras John Koenig, a Danish surgeon at Tranquebar, who had been in the service of the Nawab of Arcot. He was succeeded by Patrick Russell who collected 900 specimens, of which samples were sent to Kew for propagation. The whole collection was deposited with the Hospital Board,

> to familiarize the young Medical Gentlemen on first arrival with the principal Indian Medicinal plants which would be more generally brought into use, in preference to perishable articles now imported from England.

In 1793 Russell was succeeded as Naturalist by William Roxburgh,[2] 'the Linnaeus of Indian Botany', who had come out as Surgeon's Mate and been appointed Assistant-Surgeon at Madras in 1776. The Company always supported him on his botanical expeditions, appointing an Assistant-Surgeon to take over his duties so that he could investigate

> such Trees and other Vegetables as tend most to alleviate the distress of the Natives in times of Scarcity.

Each main Company settlement had its own botanical centre, and some surgeons set up their own gardens. In Calcutta the Botanical Gardens, founded in 1786, had a collection of three hundred plants brought in in eight years. In 1793 Roxburgh became Superintendent, and by 1831 there were 3,500 specimens. In Madras, Benjamin Heyne, Surgeon and Naturalist at Fort St. George, made collections of mineralogical and botanical specimens that were so large that some of them had to be left behind when he went home after twenty years in India. For his expeditions he needed 'a suite of forty'.

J.F. Royle, appointed Superintendent of the Botanical Garden at Saharanpur in 1823, was charged with the special duty of cultivating plants of medicinal value. For this he established a subsidiary garden at Mussoorie in the Himalayan foothills where conditions were favourable for, for example, henna, aconite, belladona, digitalis, senna, ipecacuanha and valerian. On retirement in 1837 he was appointed to the first Chair of Materia Medica at King's College, London.

These botanical collections, with their information on medicinal plants, were the basis of the first Indian pharmocopoeias (p. 251). The publication of botanical knowledge and the correspondence between interested collectors led to the formation of the first medical societies and the publication of the first medical journals. As in Europe, the scientific societies preceded the medical. The Asiatick Society, founded in 1784, was at first concerned mostly with botany and natural history (p. 150). The Medical and Physical Society of Calcutta was founded in 1823 and its *Transactions*, from 1825, was the first medical journal in India.

Much of the knowledge of medicinal herbs in the classical Indian texts had come originally from the forest dwellers and herdsmen. The physicians might live in the forest or the hills or go themselves to collect the plants at the proper time. They all learned the actions of the plants used to feed animals,[3] and the plants that animals would avoid. But there was great regional variation and there was always a problem with the identification of drugs and of the plants from which they came. Because of variations of climate in different parts of India, not all medicinal plants were available in all regions. If substitutes had to be used they might not have uniform properties. Nomenclature was another problem – the name of a plant varied from region to region, and for a popular name there might be up to twenty different plants.

Even when correctly identified, all drugs, herbal and mineral, were often found to be adulterated. Musk might be mixed with cow's liver, dried and beaten to powder. Expensive imports were often counterfeited, such as China Root, highly regarded for the treatment of syphilis. Dishonest spice-sellers would first extract the essence, and then sell the husk as the intact product. The English traders soon learned how to test to avoid fraud.

In the Hindu materia medica animal products were rare compared with vegetable. But dried lizards were still popular in the early twentieth century as they were in Europe in the sixteenth and seventeenth centuries. Some of the drugs that the early traders encountered were familiar, e.g. opium, although they commented on its widespread use and high dosage in India. Others were new to them but would be taken into medical practice when their properties had been established. New drugs were introduced from outside India, e.g.

Peruvian bark (quinine), and some old drugs were found to be particularly effective for Indian diseases, e.g. mercury.

Many of the drugs used in India came from Persia. One of the most highly valued was the bezoar stone.[4] The best stones came from Persian goats. They were strongly recommended as an antidote to poisons, and they were very scarce and costly. In India stones from the goats of Golconda were popular. Stones were also found in other animals but these were sold much more cheaply. Stones from cows had only one-fifth of the potency of the goat bezoar, but for ox bezoar they would pay 'five times its weight in silver'. Elephant bezoars were so rare that

> they are bought and hoarded up by the great and speculative Men; therefore seldom or never to be found among the Brokers in the Bazars.

Garcia da Orta (p. 25) had given the first European description of the bezoar's properties:

> it is of such use that it miraculously dilates the powers of the heart. I have had many patients who said to me after taking it, not knowing what it was, that the medicine they had eaten had given them renewed force, and made the soul return to the body. I did much good to the Bishop of Malacca, by giving him *bezar* stone with treacle.

He regarded it as the best remedy for cholera. Bontius (p. 26) recommended *lapis porcinus* from the gall-bladder of the Indian porcupine. Ambroise Paré (1582) quoted da Orta but was himself sceptical. When a nobleman presented the King with a bezoar, the King asked about its efficacy as an antidote to poison. Paré suggested a trial on a man about to be hanged. The criminal was given poison followed shortly by the bezoar. He died after seven hours of unrelieved agony. At autopsy Paré found 'the botome of his stomache blacke and dry'. He concluded that the man had been given corrosive sublimate, and that the antidote was useless.

Poisoning in the East Indies was so common and bezoars regarded as such a valuable antidote that

> any of any account keep some in their houses, and the noblemen doe horde them upp for great jewells.

The English copied this habit:

and surely I doe hold that to bee the thing, next under God, that hath preserved the moste of our lives that have been long resident there.

Bezoars were also given in fevers and as cordials – 'the Eastern Physicians prescribe this in the room of any thing else'; the stone was grated into powder, and two to three grains given in a spoonful of rose-water. The stones were commonly adulterated with wax or resin to increase the weight. This could be tested by touching with a red-hot iron – 'if they fry like Resin or Wax, they are nought.' If the surface was polished, it was always suspect, 'its Skin or Coat, when 'tis first taken out of the Body of the Animal, being Rough and Greenish'.

Their reputation lasted well into the seventeenth century. The English found that the stones were regarded highly enough to be used as presents between kings. The King of Bantam in 1606 sent two stones as a present for King James. Thomas Best, captain of the tenth voyage (1612-14), quarrelled with the Directors on his return and tried to placate them by sending a bezoar as a present. Sir Thomas Roe (p. 30) used them as presents for those he wished to impress, although he did not believe that they would protect a man from severe poisoning. He noted that

> Sir Thomas Smyth[5] is alway furnished plentifully, yet they will not cure his gowt. The less knowing People, and the Quacks, cry it up to the Skies; but in the Bottom, it is a Drug that looses its esteem in the East, and that will, in a short time, be entirely cry'd down, as I think it is already in Europe.

By the eighteenth century, although Europeans would sometimes use it medicinally, its more general use was 'like gamboge, for painters in miniature'.

A number of other stones were reputed to have medicinal properties. Snake-stones (Cobra Stone), said to be found in the heads of certain snakes, were sold by brahmins for the treatment of snake-bite (p. 95). The stone adhered to the wound until it had sucked out all the venom. Then it dropped off 'like a glutted Horse-Leach'. When placed in woman's milk it would disgorge itself and regain its power. The Archbishop of Goa had one of these stones which had cured one of his servants who had been bitten.

Goa stones were made and sold by the Jesuits in the monasteries in Goa, and brought them in a large income. There was a stone occurring in the brain of a white cow that would cure 'the falling sickness'. Rarest of all was the Magnetick Square Stone, which would deliver a woman in labour with a dead child, 'when the whole Art of Midwifery is foil'd'.

> But, one of them having been try'd by Recommendation in England,
> I find the Snake-stone and it may go together.

The English traders knew that all these stones were commonly faked, and they knew how to test if they were genuine. By the end of the seventeenth century they had all been tried out and found to be ineffective. Most of them, including the famed Cobra Stone, consisted of the ashes of the roots of plants mixed with clay or charred bone.

Pearl was often ground up and included in medicines, particularly those intended for wealthy patients, and as an antacid in diseases of the bladder:

> operating (as all Conchous things do) either by precipitating the Saline or Acid particles, or else as all Alkalies do, by imbibing the same, obtund their Fury by sheathing their sharp Points, and so render them capable of assisting such Diseases.

A pearl pendant worn by Europeans in the left ear was much admired at the Indian Courts. It was a common custom in Europe in the seventeenth century as an aid to weak sight.

Betel[6] was chewed all day by Indians, 'as commonly used as bread in Europe'. It stained the teeth red but this was one of its attractions in Indian women,[7] and

> lips remain so red, that many European Ladies would purchase it at any rate.

It had the social function of sweetening the breath — it was necessary for an inferior addressing a superior, and before making love. The Portuguese had taken to betel at once. The English were less enthusiastic although they noted that there were very few Indians with stinking breath. But some thought it was 'a vitious habit ... like tobacco'. It made 'those who are not used to it, as drunk as smoking Tabacco will do'. Toothache seemed rare in India, and this was attributed to the constant use of betel, 'and I, using it as they did, never felt that Pain, tho' otherwise subject to it'. Among its other reported medical benefits were the cure of flatulence, phlegm, worms, and the prevention of stone in the bladder. It was also an aphrodisiac and its effects could be increased by adding *ganja* (cannabis).

Opium, grown in a large and expanding tract along the Ganges, was being used all over India by the time the English arrived. By the end of the eighteenth century India was the largest supplier and China the largest consumer (p. 203). It had been introduced from West Asia by Arab traders in the twelfth century and by the Muslims as their substitute for alcohol. In Persia it was originally a sleeping draught, and for 'Men in great Places, to alay the Uneasiness of troublesome Affairs'. In India it was used to dispose of princes and some state-criminals instead of formal execution, or to incapacitate the king's children so that they would be unable to reign. Large doses, often mixed with hempseed and *nux vomica* (strychnine)

> so emaciated them by the loss of appetite that they lost their strength and intellect, and eventually died.

Indians said that this was less barbarous than killing them as they did in Turkey, or blinding them as in Persia.

Opium was used to prolong sexual intercourse although it was known that with very large doses a man would be 'unable to keep company with a woman'. A Muslim with several wives might take it before visiting them, in case the natural impulse would be so strong as to be harmful. The English did not regard opium as particularly dangerous,[8] and many of them took small doses with their meals to strengthen their nerves and promote digestion: 'it relieved tension in the nerves – essential in a hot climate.' Army officers, in particular, used it frequently. Many Europeans in India became addicted.[9] Most European women in India, exhausted by the heat, needed wet-nurses for their children. These nurses, as was the Indian custom, gave the children opium to make them sleep, and it is thought that many children may have died from this habit. It was widely prescribed by Hindu practitioners for pain and sleep. The English soon noted that Indians took it in doses that would have killed a European, and that the effects were more deadly than alcohol. Starting with a pill the size of a pinhead they gradually increased the dose up to the size of a pea. The soldiers fought well on it but they became unfit at an early age. It helped workers in harsh conditions. Messengers took it to increase their endurance and to relieve hunger. The Rajputs, the most valiant fighters of all the Hindus, were accustomed to it from an early age:

> On the day of battle they never fail to double the dose, and this drug so animates them, or rather inebriates them, that they rush into the thickest of the combat insensible of dangers.

With very large doses they were liable to run amok and attack friend as well as foe. The opium addicts in the general population were crippled with pains in their bones, and they never reached old age.

Among other narcotics, Indian hemp[10] was used 'to provoke lust'. It was used freely by Muslims, but was forbidden to some sects of Hindus:

> by Reason of its pernicious Effects on the Brain; But in all Sects, none but the Scum of the People drink of it, especially the Mumpers [beggars]; they never miss taking it once a day, except upon a journey, for then they take it three or four times a day, and by the Virtue of that Drink, they walk more Briskly and Nimbly ... the use of it becomes Mortal in Time, like that of Opium.

It enabled a man to carry out heavy work without fatigue and was much used by slaves and soldiers before a battle. On forced marches by English troops the commanding officer might order cannabis or a double ration of spirits.

Datura, 'a kind of Stramonea',[11] deprived a man of his senses even though his eyes remained open. It was used by wandering gangs of robbers to immobilize their victims. Women also found it useful in hiding their illicit affairs from their husbands. The man could always be revived by cold water to the soles of his feet.

Before the introduction of inhalation anaesthesia in the middle of the nineteenth century, various combinations of these narcotics, often with 'a fair dose of wine', were used to relieve the pain of operations.

Cinchona bark (Peruvian/Spanish bark, with its most important alkaloid, quinine) reached Europe in the middle of the seventeenth century. Named after the Countess of Cinchon, wife of the Spanish Viceroy in Lima in 1638, who was the first European to be cured of malaria, it was sent to Rome by Jesuits in Peru. The bark was imported into England from Antwerp. But it was suspect because it had been introduced by the Jesuits. It was so effective that it was thought that they must have charmed it or even invoked the Devil to help them. No good Protestant physician would prescribe it until Thomas Sydenham (p. 81) wrote of its value in 1676. The next year it was included in the London Pharmacopoeia. Given powdered it was known as Countess's or Jesuit's powder. It was very bitter, so that patients would refuse to take it unless it was made up into a tincture in wine.

The bark was expensive and there were many substitutes, which gave rise to reports that batches of the bark had lost their effect. It was commonly adulterated so that double doses had to be given. Confusion between the types of fever also cast doubt on its efficacy although the dramatic response of 'malarial' fevers helped in the differentiation.[12] In India it was used not only for fevers but also for abscesses, wounds, colic and snake-bite. Up to the early nineteenth century the crude bark was used. From 1815 there was a start on separating out its different components. The supply from Peru was endangered by careless collection and reckless destruction of many trees. In 1854 the Dutch brought specimens of bark and planted them in Java. The British set up plantations in Ceylon and India but the Dutch had the better stock and gradually got the monopoly. In the twentieth century 80 per cent of the world's supplies came from the East Indies and the rest from India, while it had almost disappeared from Peru.

Mercury had long been known as the most effective remedy for syphilis. All the traders brought large supplies with them, but, as well as treating venereal disease, they found that mercury seemed to have a specific effect on some Indian diseases. The general opinion that all diseases in India had a common cause – the climate – meant that they could all be treated in more or less the same way. Both patients and doctors had faith in mercury which was given, sometimes in massive doses, for most of the common disorders. The medical Indent for 1789 for Madras included 'one thousand Pounds weight of Quicksilver exclusive of the usual Proportions of the different Mercurial preparations'. Its mode of action was unknown but it seemed a panacea, as though it 'induced a state in the system totally opposite to disease'. It was credited with almost magical properties. There are frequent references to 'being under the protection of mercury' and 'not being safe until under its influence'. If the patient was taking mercury (most commonly for venereal disease) he was less liable to fever, even in the most dangerous seasons.

In many cases when salivation (ptyalism) and a sore mouth (the tests of a satisfactory dose) had been induced, they could be continued for weeks with no apparent serious injury. Mercury could therefore be safely prescribed for every minor affection of the digestive system, for rheumatism, and even for mental disease and as a tonic. If it failed it was the fault of the climate. In extreme heat it might be difficult to affect the mouth to salivation, and this was thought to be an indication for increasing the dose. Indian dressers were employed to carry out frictions with mercury ointment for hours at a time. To increase the absorption, delicate areas of skin were treated – between the fingers and in the armpit and groin – having first had their surface layers removed by blistering.

By the second quarter of the nineteenth century some surgeons in India were protesting at the excessive mercurialization that was the standard practice in most diseases. It was recognized that mercury was a powerful remedy for tropical diseases, but there was still not enough investigation to allow its rational use. All that was known (as shown by experiments on dogs) was that it stimulated the secretion of bile by the liver. But it was not clear even if and when this was necessary. When treating Indians it was found that all fluxes got worse with mercury; the patients were susceptible to every sort of intercurrent infection and the mortality was very high. The same applied to Europeans on a strictly vegetable diet. If calomel (mercurous chloride) was used at all, it should be in small doses and intended simply as a purge.

There was also a reaction in England to the widespread use of mercury. The reports of its successes in India had encouraged over-use in England where it was tried for every 'bilious' disorder. There had always been some abuse by quacks offering it as a cure-all. But now, in the form of calomel, it was taking the place of magnesia in nurseries, and was a constituent of popular remedies for worms and diseases of the skin such as ringworm. It was realized that too much attention had been given to Indian diseases although it was clear that mercury was as specific for 'hepatitis' in India as for syphilis (p. 89). Even in venereal disease, where mercury was the only hope of cure, it was now recognized that some of the symptoms and some of the destruction of tissue were due to the treatment and not to the disease. But often the complications were still thought to be venereal so that more mercury was given.

Although the harmful effects of mercury were not noted in some of the contemporary text-books, the 'mercurial disease' was becoming less common in Britain. But there were still patients with 'inordinate ptyalism', ulcerations and pains in the bones. This over-dosing was thought to be due to the inexperience of the practitioner, often a young surgeon treating venereal disease, and was attributed to

> a most unaccountable and general opinion, that the administration of mercury was the department of the surgeon, and hence its use was freely exercised by many juniors in the profession, to the exclusion of the more aged and experienced.

In India, there were frequent reports of the complications of mercury, which had been prescribed not only by Europeans but also by Indian practitioners who were particularly liable to overuse it. There were patients with intractable pain and swelling of the limbs, loss of hearing and memory, nervous complaints, and some whose noses and faces had been destroyed.[13] It was particularly dangerous in scurvy, leading to increased ulceration. But the sore gums in scurvy had to be differentiated from an overdose of mercury, as so many of the patients were already on calomel for syphilis. It was wrong to teach that

> where mercury is useful, the mouth must be made sore, and that, when the mouth is sore, the patient may be considered safe.

In some patients it was impossible to make the mouth sore, and to continue would be dangerous. But, in spite of the debate both in Europe and in India, no investigations were made of the direct effects of mercury.

Mummy (mumia) from bodies that had been preserved in dry soil for two thousand years had always been valued by the Arabs, and later in Europe, for its medicinal properties. The demand produced many fakes until these were exposed at the end of the sixteenth century. There was also a Persian variety[14] obtained from a cave in the mountains. It all belonged to the King, who distributed it as a mark of favour. Europeans trading with Persia heard of its miraculous healing powers in man and animals:

> let a human body be never so much mill'd, broken, torn and even minced all to pieces, one half Drachm of this Mummy will re-establish it in four and twenty Hours time.

Animal fat was, for Europeans, an important ingredient of medicaments, and there were new and effective varieties in the East. Crocodile fat was 'very good for several operations in Physick and Surgery'. Elephant fat could be rubbed in to strengthen weak sinews, and the hide and toe-nails, with stag's horn, were used to fumigate piles and inflammations.

Human fat, recommended particularly for nervous disorders and contractures of the joints, was collected from the bodies of criminals who had been well fed for a month before execution and were then hung over an open fire under the gibbet. No other 'animal' fat was used in Hindu medicaments.

Cow-dung and urine had purifying virtues for Hindus. Smearing the walls and floors of houses with cow-dung would remove pollution by a Christian. It gave a smooth surface which kept vermin away and protected against plague. Sins could be cleansed by eating cow-dung in urine with butter and sour milk. This was an essential part of the purification process for Hindus who had converted to Islam, or who had been taken prisoner by Muslims or Christians. For the first six months after returning to the fold they were required 'to mix amongst what they are to eat, a pound of Cow-dung'. In their fasts, they would take only 'the fresh Stale of the Worshipful Cow', which was also valuable for its purging and cleansing properties. Europeans were advised to use this remedy to regain their health after frequent bleedings, particularly as practised by the Portuguese. Three glasses of cow's urine were prescribed daily for twelve days. Most of the convalescents found the remedy so unpleasant that they took as little of it as possible, however keen they were to regain their strength.

Tobacco was introduced into India about the end of the sixteenth century. The habit spread steadily in spite of opposition by the authorities. The English were familiar with the medicinal properties of tobacco as an infusion for inflammations and poisonous bites. It was also given as an enema for the reduction of a strangulated hernia but this was later abandoned as it could prove fatal.

Muslims were never without their hookahs,[15] even on horseback. They agreed that it was weakening but life had no joy without it. The British adopted the custom with enthusiasm – ' a day and night addiction' (p. 104). The water had to be changed at least once a day as it became very rank and was then used as 'a great Emetick, and would almost make a Man Vomit his Heart up'. Only the lowest classes, European and Indian, smoked cheroots. The hookah continued into the nineteenth century when it was replaced by the cigar.

Tea was already well-known for its health-giving properties, and was used all over India as well as by the English and the Dutch to cleanse the stomach and by its 'temperate heat to digest the superfluous humours'. Indians added spice and sugar-candy or 'Syrrop of Limons', and took it for 'Head-Ach, Gravel and Griping of the Gut'.

Coffee was also used to maintain health by helping digestion, lifting the spirits and cleansing the blood. It was not grown in India but was imported, mainly by the Dutch, from Mocca. In India strict abstainers from wine would drink coffee.

Sugar had always been known in India, although it was generally believed that 'the Ancients us'd nothing but Honey'. It was plentiful in Bengal in the seventeenth century. Much of the honey was not collected because Hindus would not destroy life to get the combs.

Spices were also used medicinally but they were generally expensive. Cardamom was very scarce, and was only used by nobles; it cost four times as much as pepper which was one of the most lucrative of the Company's cargoes. Tamarind, the Indian date, was regarded as the best sauce for all curries but it was also a good purge and cheap so that it was the common remedy of the poor.

Musk was much used for perfumes and aphrodisiacs, and

> the women make use of it to dissipate the Vapours, which rise from the Matrix into the Brain ... applying it to the Part, which modesty will not permit me to name.

Henna was used by women to decorate their palms and soles. It was astringent, used to check perspiration and to 'correct the scent of the habitual discharge from the feet' (although there was some doubt whether it was always wise to obstruct this). The English noticed that it was very rare in Indians because of their frequent washing.

Pepper was valued for its cooling properties, and used copiously in congee (rice-water) in high fevers.

Delicious fruit and vegetables were available in profusion but over-indulgence could cause a flux that was more severe than in temperate climates. Eating too many dates, when not accustomed to them, could heat the blood, cause ulcers all over the body, and weaken the sight, although the local inhabitants were never affected in this way. Apricots were known to the locals as 'kill-Franks' [*firenghi* – foreigner]. But fruit could also relieve disease. Mangoes were not only delicious, but also medically recommended – 'the gentlemen eat little else in the hot months', and 'if no wine is drank with them, they are apt to throw out troublesome but healthful boils.' Boiled mango was an infallible remedy for the flux. Melon was a remedy for all distempers, taken in vast amounts in April to purge and cool the blood although it was recognized that such excess could cause fevers.

By 1840 Ainslie, Royle and others felt that, as a result of the work of the Company surgeon-botanists, all that was of value of the materia medica of India had been collected and recorded. Whitelaw Ainslie had first written about this in 1813, and his enlarged edition (1826) became the standard for nearly 50 years. In the *Bengal Dispensatory* (1842) William O'Shaughnessy, professor of chemistry at the Bengal Medical College, was the first to subject indigenous drugs to chemical analysis. Each Presidency published its own pharmacopoeia: Bengal 1844, Madras 1855 and Bombay 1862. The combined material was the basis of the first official *Pharmacopoeia of India* in 1868 edited by E.J. Waring with a committee appointed by the Secretary of State for India. This contained all the information in the *British Pharmacopoeia* of practical use in India, together with all the local products that had proved to be of value from vegetable, inorganic and animal sources.

Notes

1 In 1664 the Royal Society had set up a committee to study the transmission of plants from the East and the cultivation of spices and drugs. The collections, in eight books, were passed to Sir Hans Sloane, and now form part of the herbarium of the British Museum.

2 Roxburgh published *Plants of the Coast of Coromandel* (1795-1819), *Horten Bengalensis* (1814) and *Flora Indica*. with additions by Wallich, a Danish surgeon (1820-4).

3 Some of the grasses used to feed cattle were found to promote urination and lactation. There are now popular drugs for these functions in humans using combinations of these grasses.

4 *be-zaer*, 'conqueror of poison' (Pers.), found in the stomach of various animals, having the consistency of soft stone, with a piece of straw or wood at the centre, round which the material is deposited in coats like an onion.

5 The first Governor of the East India Company.

6 beetle, betel, pan, pawn – made from a mixture of areca-nut and lime from shells wrapped in the leaf (pan) of *piper betel*.

7 Since the despised dogs and monkeys have white teeth, black or discoloured teeth were regarded as beautiful.

8 Opium and its many preparations were on open sale in England with widespread medical and social use until restricted by the Pharmacy Act of 1868.

9 Robert Clive, towards the end of his life in 1787, was taking fifteen grains a day.

10 Bhang, buing, hashish, cannabis.

11 Thorn-apple.

12 Malaria was not separated from other fevers until the nineteenth century. Quinine was not used prophylactically until about 1840,

13 The first 'Indian' operation in Europe (1814) was on an army officer whose nose had been destroyed by over-use of mercury for a liver complaint (p. 173).

14 Probably bitumen or 'Jew's pitch' – the term mummy deriving from the preservation of lower-class bodies in pitch.

15 *hukkah*, a round casket (Arabic). A mixture of tobacco, sweet herbs, sugar and spices, smoked through rose-water. Indians often added hashish or opium.

BIBLIOGRAPHY

Preface

Medical systems
Goodeve, H. H. 'A sketch of the progress of European Medicine in the East', *Quart. J. Calc. Med. Phys. Soc.* 2 124 1837
Leslie, C. ed. *Asian Medical Systems: a comparative study* U. Cal. Press 1976
Roy, K. K. 'Early relations between the British and Indian medical systems', *Proc. XXIII Int. Congr. Hist. Med.* I 697 1974
Subba Reddy, D. V. *The Beginnings of Modern Medicine in Madras* Calcutta 1947
----- 'Medical literature in India, ancient, mediaeval and modern', *Ann. Ind. Acad. Med. Sci.* 9 1 1975

Social interaction
Carey, W. H. *The Good Old Days of Honourable John Company 1600-1858* Calcutta 1906
Iyer, R. ed. *The Glass Curtain between Asia and Europe. A Symposium on the historical encounters and the changing attitudes of the peoples of the East and West* London 1965
Moorhouse, G. *India Britannica* London 1983
Mudford, P. *Birds of a different plumage. A study of British-Indian relations from Akbar to Curzon* London 1974
Wilkinson, T. *Two Monsoons* London 1976
Yule, H. and Burnell, A. C. *Hobson-Jobson. A glossary of colloquial Anglo-Indian words and phrases and of kindred terms, etymological, historical, geographical and discursive* (1886) reprinted London 1986
Yusuf Ali, A. *A Cultural History of India during the British Period* Bombay 1940

Chapter 1

Panikkar, K. M. *Malabar and the Portuguese* Bombay 1929
Pinkerton, J. *A general collection of the best and most interesting Voyages and Travels to all parts of the World* London 1811-12
Radwan, A. B. *The Dutch in Western India 1601-1632* Calcutta 1978

Stevens, H. *The dawn of British Trade to the East Indies as recorded in the Court Minutes of the East India Company (1599-1603)* London 1886
Wheeler, J. T. *Early Travels in India* Calcutta 1864

Chapter 2

General

Basham, A. L. 'The Practice of Medicine in Ancient and Medieval India' in *Asian Medical Systems* ed. C. Leslie, U. Cal. Press 1976
Bose, D. M., Sen, S. N. and Subbarayappa, B. V. *A concise history of science in India* New Delhi 1971
Jaggi, O. P. *History of Science and Technology in India* Delhi 1973
Patterson, T. J. S. 'Science and Medicine in India', in *Information Sources in the History of Science and Medicine* ed. P. Weindling and P. Corsi, London 1983
----- 'The relationship of Indian and European practitioners of medicine from the sixteenth century', in *Studies on Indian Medical History* ed. G. J. Meulenbeld and D. Wujastyk, Groningen 1987
Subba Reddy, D. V. 'Medicine in India in the middle of the XVI century', *Bull. Hist. Med.* 8 40 1940

Ayurveda

Filliozat, J. *The Classical Doctrine of Indian Medicine, its origins and its Greek parallels* (Paris 1949), transl. D. R. Chanana, Delhi 1964
Ray, P. 'Origin and tradition of alchemy', *Ind. J. Hist. Med.* 2 1 1967
Ray, P. and Gupta, H. N. *Caraka Samhita (a scientific synopsis)* New Delhi 1965
----- and Roy, M. *Susruta Samhita (a scientific synopsis)* New Delhi 1980
Singhal, G. D. and Patterson, T. J. S. *Synopsis of Ayurveda, based on a translation of the Susruta Samhita* New Delhi 1993
Wujastyk, D. *The Roots of Ayurveda* Penguin Books India 1998

Siddha

Kutumbiah, P. 'The Siddha and Rasa Sidha Schools of Indian medicine', *Ind. J. Hist. Med.* 18 21 1973
Subba Reddy, D. V. 'History of Siddha Medicine', *Bull. Inst. Hist. Med. 3* 182 1973

Unani

Browne, E. G. *Arabian Medicine* Cambridge 1962
Dols, M. *Medieval Islamic Medicine* U. Cal. Press 1964
Siddiqui, M. Z. 'The *Unani tibb* (Greek Medicine in India)', in Bose, Sen

and Subbarayappa, New Delhi 1971
Verma, R. L. 'The growth of Greco-Arabian medicine in medieval India', *Ind. J. Hist. Sci.* 5 347 1970

Chapter 3

The Company
Birdwood, G. and Foster W. *The Register of Letters etc. of the Governour and Company of Merchants of London trading into the East Indies 1600-1619* London 1893
Crawford, D. G. *A History of the Indian Medical Service 1600-1913* London 1914
Gardner, R. B, *The East India Company. A History* London 1971
Keay, J. *The Honourable Company. A History of the English East India Company* London 1991
McDonald, D. *Surgeons Twoe and a Barber. Being some account of the life and work of the Indian Medical Service (1600-1947)* London 1950
Mukherjee, R. *The Rise and Fall of the East India Company* New York 1974
Wheeler, J. T. *Early Records of British India* London 1878
Willson, B. *Ledger and Sword, or The Honourable Company of Merchants of England Trading to the East Indies (1599-1874)* London 1903

The Surgeons
Cheevers, N. 'Surgeons in India — Past and Present', *Calcutta Review* 23 217 1854
Keynes, G. 'John Woodall, surgeon, his place in medical history', *J. Roy. Coll. Phys. Lond.* 2 15 1967
Woodall, J. *The Surgions Mate* London 1617 (facs. J. Kirkup, Bath, 1976)

Their knowledge of India
Lach, D. F. *India in the eyes of Europe. The sixteenth century* U. Chic. Press 1968
Linschoten, J. *The Voyage of John Huyghen van Linschoten to the East Indies* (English translation 1598) ed. A. C. Burnell and P. A. Tiele for the Haklyut Society, London 1885
Neelameghan, A. 'The Royal Hospital at Goa as described in some seventeenth century travel accounts', *Ind. J. Hist. Med.* 6 52 1961
da Orta, G. *Coloquios dos simples e drogas he cousas medicinais da India* (Goa 1563) transl. G. Markham,
The simples and drugs of India London 1913
Pyrard de Laval *The Voyage of Francois Pyrard de Laval to the East Indies, the Maldives, the Moluccas and Brazil* (English translation 1619) ed. A.

Gray for the Hakluyt Society, London 1890

Wateson, G. *The Cures of the Diseased, in remote Regions. Preventing mortalitie, incident in Forraine Attempts of the English Nation* London 1598 (facs. ed. C. Singer Oxford 1915)

Chapter 4

Voyages

Best, T. *The Voyage of Thomas Best to the East Indies 1612-14* ed. W. Foster for the Haklyut Society, London 1934

Downton, N. *The voyage of Nicholas Downton to the East Indies 1614-15* ed. W. Foster for the Hakluyt Society, London 1939

Floris, P. *His voyage to the East Indies in the Globe 1611-1615* ed. W. H. Moreland for the Hakluyt Society, London 1934

Jourdain, J. *The Journal of John Jourdain 1608-1617, describing his experiences in Arabia, India and the Malay Archipelago* ed. W. Foster for the Hakluyt Society, Cambridge 1905

Lancaster, J. *The Voyages of Sir James Lancaster to Brazil and the East Indies 1591-1603* ed. W. Foster for the Hakluyt Society London 1940

Middleton, H. *The Voyage of Sir Henry Middleton to the Moluccas 1604-6* ed. W. Foster for the Hakluyt Society, London 1943

Saris, J. *The Voyage of Captain John Saris to Japan 1613* ed. E. M. Satow for the Hakluyt Society, London 1900

Camoëns, Luis de *The Lusiad; or, the discovery of India* (1572) tr. W. J. Mickie, 3 ed. London 1798

Milton, G. *Nathaniel's Nutmeg* London 1999 [the Massacre at Amboyna]

Roe, T. *The Embassy of Sir Thomas Roe to the Court of the Great Mogul 1615-18* ed. W. Foster for the Hakluyt Society, London 1899

Strachan, M. *Sir Thomas Roe 1581-1644* Salisbury 1989

Tickner, F. J. and Medvei, V. C. 'Scurvy and the health of European crews in the Indian Ocean in the seventeenth century', *Med. Hist. 36* 1958

Chapter 5

Despatches from England 1670-77
Diary and Consultation Book Madras 1672-78
Factory Records, Fort St. George 1647
Fort St. David Consultations 1696

Methwold, W. *Relations of Golconda in the early seventeenth century* ed. W. H. Moreland, for the Hakluyt Society, London 1931

Subba Reddy, D. V. 'Medicine at the Moghul Court', *J. Ind. Hist.* **17** 165 1938
----- 'Medical relief in mediaeval South India', *Bull. Hist. Med.* **9** 385 1941
Terry, E. *A Voyage to East-India; wherein Some Things are taken Notice of, in our Passage Thither, But Many More in our Abode There within that Rich and most Spacious Empire of the Great Mogul* reprinted from the edition of 1655, London 1777

Chapter 6

Bernier, Francois *Travels in the Mogul Empire AD 1656-1668* (1670)
    transl. A. Constable (1891); 2nd. ed. V. A. Smith, London 1914
Crawford, D. G. 'The Legend of Gabriel Boughton', *Ind. Med. Gaz.* Jan. 1907
Manucci, N. *Storia do Mogor* Venice 1653-1708 transl. W. Irvine London 1907
Marshall, J. 'A letter from the East Indies of Mr John Marshall', *Phil. Trans.* **22**, 729 1700-01
----- *John Marshall in India. Notes and Observations in Bengal 1668-1672*
    ed. S. A. Khan, London 1927
Mundy, P. *The Travels of Peter Mundy, in Europe and Asia 1608-1638*
    ed. Carnac Temple for the Hakluyt Society, Cambridge 1907-1919

Chapter 7

Travellers
Barlow, E. *Barlow's Journal of his life at sea in King's Ships, East and West Indiamen and other merchantmen from 1659 to 1703* ed. B. Lubbock, London 1934
Chardin, J. *The Travels of Sir John Chardin into Persia and the East-Indies* (translated under the author's supervision) London 1686
Ovington, J. *A Voyage to Suratt, in the Year 1689* London 1696
Tavernier, J. B. *Travels in India* (1676) tr. V. Ball, London 1889
Thevenot, J, de *Collected travels* (Paris 1664-1684) London 1687
----- *Indian travels of Thevenot and Careri* ed. S. Sen New Delhi 1949

Medical
Dellon, C. [physician] *A Voyage to the East Indies* (Paris 1684-5) transl. J. Krull London 1698
Fryer, G. 'John Fryer, F. R. S. and his scientific observations, made chiefly in India and Persia between 1672 and 1682', *Notes and Records of the Royal Society of London* **33** 175 1979
Fryer, J. *A new Account of East India and Persia, being Nine Years Travels, 1672-1681* London 1698

Kennedy, R. H. 'On Dracunculus', *Trans. Med. Phys. Soc. Calc. 1* 151 1825
Ramana Rao, V. V. 'Indian Goddesses in Epidemic Diseases' [smallpox] *Bull. Inst. Hist. Med. 1* 44 1971
Subba Reddy, D. V. An Account of Indian Medicine by John Fryer *Ind.Med. Gaz.* Jan. 35 1940
Twining, W. 'Ipecacuanha in dysentery', *Trans. Med. Phys. Soc. Calc. 4* 170 1829
Wilson, H. H. 'On the native practice in cholera', *Trans. Med. Phys. Soc. Calc. 2* 202 1826

Chapter 8

Crawford, D. G. 'William Hamilton and the Embassy to Delhi', *Ind. Med. Gaz.* Jan. 1909.
Pillai, A. R. *The private diary of Ananda Ranga Pillai* ed. J. F. Price, Madras 1904
Spear, P. *The Nabobs. A study of the social life of the English in eighteenth century India* London 1963
----- *Master of Bengal. Clive and his India* London 1975

Travellers
Grose, J. H. *A Voyage to the East-Indies: began in 1750,* London 1766
Hamilton, A. *A new Account of the East Indies... from the Year 1688 to 1723* Edinburgh 1727
Kindersley, Mrs. J. *Letters from the Island of Teneriffe, Brazil, The Cape of Good Hope, and the East Indies* London 1777
Symson, W. *A New Voyage to the East Indies* London 1720

Medical
Clark, J. *Observations on the Diseases which prevail in long Voyages to Hot Countries, particularly on those in the East Indies* Edinburgh 1792
Ives, E. [surgeon] *A Voyage from England to India in the Year MDCCLIV.* London 1773
Lind, J. *A Treatise of the Scurvy* Edinburgh 1753
----- *An Essay on Diseases incidental to Europeans in hot Climates* London 1768
Pringle, J. *Observations on the diseases of the Army* London 1752

Chapter 9

Cotton, E. and Fawcett, C. *East Indiamen. The East India Company's Maritime Service* London 1949
Fryke, C. and Schewitzer, C. *A Relation of Two several Voyages made into the East-Indies* London 1700

Medical
Balfour, F. *A Treatise on the Action of Sol-Lunar Influence* Edinburgh 1791
Blane, G. *The diseases of seamen* London 1785

Curtis, C. *An Account of the Diseases of India, as they appeared in the English Fleet, and in the Naval Hospital at Madras, in 1782* Edinburgh and London 1807

Dharampal, *Indian Science and Technology in the Eighteenth Century* Delhi 1971

Geddes, J. L. 'Remarks on Malignant Ulcer and Hospital Gangrene', *Trans. Med. Phys. Soc. Calc.* 6   147   1833

Loudon, I. S. L. 'Leg ulcers in the eighteenth and early nineteenth centuries', *J. Roy. Coll. Gen. Pract.* 31 263 1981

Williams, J. 'On the Cure of Persons bitten by Snakes', *Asiatick Researches 2* 323   1790

Chapter 10

Medical Board Proceedings Calcutta
Surgeon General's Records Madras
Hospital Board Records Bombay

Cannon, G. *Oriental Jones* Bombay 1964

Sen, S. N. 'Scientific Works in Sanskrit, translated into foreign languages and vice versa in the 18th and 19th Century AD', *Ind. J. Hist. Sci.* 7 44 1972

Medical

Ernst, W. 'The establishment of Native Lunatic Asylums in early nineteenth century British India', in *Studies on Indian Medical History*, ed. G. J. Meulenbeld and D. Wujastyk, Groningen   1987

Hunter, W. W. *Annals of rural Bengal* London   1868 [the famine of 1770].

Hutchinson, J. *A Report on the Medical Management of the Native Jails* Calcutta   1837

Chapter 11

Williamson, T. *The East India Vade-Mecum; or, Complete Guide to Gentlemen intended for the Civil, Military, or Naval Service of the Hon. East India Company* London 1810

Basu, R. N., Jezek, Z. and Ward, N. A. *The Eradication of Smallpox from India* New Delhi 1979

Bell, W. 'On lithotomy', *Trans. Med. Soc. Calc.* 6   455 1833

Breton, P. 'On the Native Mode of Couching', *Trans. Med. Soc.. Calc.* 2 342 1826

Carpue, J. C. *An Account of Two Successful Operations for restoring a lost Nose*

from the Integuments of the Forehead London 1816
Keegan, D. F. *Rhinoplastic Operations* London 1900
Raleigh, W. W. 'Modification of the Oriental operation of Couching' *Trans. Med. Phys. Soc. Calc.* 6 137 1833
Twining, W, 'On the effects of blood-letting in the cold stage of intermittent fevers', *Trans. Med. Phys. Soc. Calc.* 5 58 1831
Wilson, H. H. '*Kushta,* or Leprosy, as known to the Hindus', *Trans. Med. Phys. Soc. Calc.* 1 1 1825

Chapter 12

Burnes, J. *A narrative of a visit to the Court of Sinde* Bombay 1829
Forbes, J. *Oriental Memoirs: a Narrative of seventeen years residence in India* London 1834
Wise, T. A. *Commentary on the Hindu System of Medicine* London 1845

Education
Eatwell, W. C. B. *On the rise and progress of rational medical education in Bengal* Calcutta 1860
Neelameghan, A. *Development of medical societies and medical periodicals in India, 1780 to 1920* Calcutta 1963
Sarbadadhikari, K. C. 'Western Medical Education in India during the early days of British occupation', *Ind. J. Med. Educ.* 1 27 1961
Sen, S. N. 'The character of the introduction of western science in India during the eighteenth and the nineteenth centuries', *Ind. J. Hist. Sci.* 1 112 1966
Shryock, R. H. *The development of modern medicine* U. Wisconsin Press 1937

Public Health
Hardie, D. 'On the Malaria, and Medical Topography of Oudypoor', *Trans. Med. Phys. Soc. Calc.* 5 1 1831
Heyne, B. *Tracts, historical and statistical* London 1814
Marshall, T. 'A statistical account of the Pergunna of Jumboosur', *Trans. Lit. Soc. Bombay* 3 383 1833
Ranken, J. 'On public health in India', *Trans. Med. Phys. Soc. Calc.* 3 300 1827
Rankine, R. *Notes on the medical topography of the district of Sarun* Calcutta 1839

Medical
Annesley, J. *Sketches of the most prevalent diseases of India* London 1825
Brett, F. H. 'On Acupuncturation for cure of Chronic Rheumatism in Natives', *Trans. Med. Phys. Soc. Calc.* 5 443 1831

Chisholm, C. *A Manual of the Climate and Diseases of Tropical Countries ... a guide to the young medical practitioner on his first resorting to those countries* London 1822

Fayrer, J. *Clinical Surgery in India* London 1866

Geddes, W. 'On abscess of the liver in European subjects at the Madras Presidency', *Trans. Med. Phys. Soc. Calc.* 6 284 1833

Johnson, J. *The influence of tropical climates, more especially the climate of India on European constitutions* London 1815; 6th. ed. with J. R. Martin 1841

Mouat, J. 'Case of Beri Beri with pathological remarks', *Trans. Med. Phys. Soc. Calc.* 7 243 1835

Ross, T. 'An account of the Scurvy, which appeared in the 4th Regt. Light Cavalry at Nusserabad', *Trans. Med. Phys. Soc. Calc.* 8 130 1836

Smith, H. 'Reports on medical and surgical practice in the Jullundur Civil Hospital, Punjab', *Brit. Med. J.* 2 1180 1897

Twining, W. *Clinical illustrations of the more important Diseases of Bengal* Calcutta 1832

Chapter 13

Froggat, P. 'The East India Company (London Establishment)' *Trans. Soc. Occup. Med.* 18 111 1968

Gilchrist, J. B. *The General East India Guide and Vade Mecum, for the public functionary, Government officer, private agent, trader or foreign sojourner in British India* London 1825

Herklots, G. A. *Customs of the Moosulmans of India* London 1832

The Mutiny
Acharya, A. M. 'The First Indian War of Independence and military surgery', *Bull. Ind. Inst. Hist. Med.* 5 225 1975

Williamson, G. *Notes on the wounded from the Mutiny in India* London 1859

Further reading
Farrell, J. G. *The Siege of Krishnapur* London 1973

Hibbert, C. *The Great Mutiny. India 1857* London 1978

Chapter 14

Balfour, M. I. and Young, R. *The work of medical women in India* London 1929

Jeffery, R. *The politics of health in India* U. Cal, Press 1988

Subba Reddy, D. V. 'Dr. Mahendra Lal Sircar, the first eminent allopath to practise and propagate homoeopathy', *Bull. Inst. Hist. Med.* 4 32 1974

Chapter 15

Hehir, P. *The Medical Profession in India* London 1923
Honigberger, J. M. *Thirty-five years in the East* London 1852
Jaggi, O. P. 'Indigenous systems of Medicine during British supremacy in India', *Stud. Hist. Med.* Dec. 1977

Chapter 16

Bhatia, J. R. 'Preventive and Social Medicine failure', *Ind. J. Med. Educ. 12* 21 1973
Seal, S. C. 'A short history of public health in India', *Ind. J. Hist. Med. 15* 25 1971

Appendix

Ainslie, Whitelaw *Materia indica, or some account to those articles which are employed by the Hindoos, and other Eastern nations, in their medicine, arts, and agriculture* London 1826
Crawford, D. G. 'Famous botanists in the I.M.S.', *Ind. Med. Gaz.* 1912
Fleming, J. 'A catalogue of Indian medicinal Plants and Drugs with their Names in the Hindustani and Sanskrit Languages', *Asiatick Researches* 11 1812
Jones, W. 'On the plants of India', in *Dissertations and Miscellaneous Pieces* Calcutta 1792
Petiver, J. 'An account of some Indian plants', *Phil. Trans. 20* 313 1698
Sharma, A. L., Seerwani, A. B. and Shastry, V. R. 'Botany in the Vedas', *Ind. J. Hist. Sci. 7* 38 1972
Subba Reddy, D. V. 'Dr Samuel Browne, Physican and Proprietor of Madras in the 17th century', *Journal of the Madras University 12* 84 1941
----- 'Medical observations of Dr. Edward Ives. A Naval surgeon', *Ind. J. Hist. Med. 13* 32 1968

INDEX

Achin (Sumatra) 2, 29
acupuncture 11, 196
Afghan:
    invasion 101
    War 185
ague *see* fevers
Ainslie, Whitelaw 251
Aix la Chapelle, Peace of 101
Akbar, Emperor 11, 14, 41 (f.n.l), 43, 51
Albucasis 6
alchemy 8, 12, 82, 181 (f.n.4), 189
alcohol 49, 64, 134, 155
    in Ayurveda 8, 9, 50
    Unani 10
    Muslim drinking 10, 44, 51, 67
    medicinal 22, 39, 52, 67, 87, 97, 115-6, 121, 134-5
    at sea 39, 134
    Hindu abstinence praised 45
    health hazards 51, 52, 62, 66, 134, 155, 163, 205
    see also arrack, punch, shrub, toddy
All-India Mahasammalan 225
allopathy 8
alum 133
Amboyna, Massacre at 31
ammonia 95
amoebic dysentery *see* dysentery
anaesthesia 9, 10, 246
    see also mesmerism
anatomy, in Ayurveda 7
    Galen corrected 22
    criticism of Indian 81, 112
    first human dissection by a Hindu 200
Anderson, Dr James 125 (f.n.13), 139, 176
Anglo-Indians 130, 200, 208
animal hospitals 12, 13, 43, 55, 112
Annesley, (Sir) James 99 (f.n.11), 189
aphrodisiacs 8, 45, 84, 113, 130, 234, 244, 245, 250
apoplexy *see* heat-stroke

apricots 251
Arabs 1, 2, 3, 11, 13
Arcot, Nawab of 121, 240
    Siege of 101
arrack (arak, racke) 35, 51, 52, 66, 115, 155
arsenic 139, 181 (f.n.4)
artemesia 197
Ascension 38, 113
Asiatick Society 150, 241
Ashoka, Emperor 11, 12, 237
astrology 23, 82, 170
astronomy 152
aub-dar 129, 133
Aurangzeb, Emperor 11, 60, 67, 77, 78, 101, 171, 220
Avicenna (Ibn Sina) 6, 24, 179
Ayurveda ix, 3, 5, 6, 24, 25, 56, 61, 82, 93, 97, 104, 121, 187, 199, 200, 225, 241
    compared to European medicine 3, 13, 14, 57, 63, 149, 167
    training 7
    medical treatment 8-9
    prognosis 8, 111, 227
    surgery 9-10, 11
    influence of Buddhism 11
    compared to Unani 11
    compared to Greek 13
    animal hospitals 55
    treatment by fasting 56, 81, 87, 89, 168
    cooling for fevers 80, 87, 193
    criticism of 80, 81, 82, 111-2, 167, 170, 186, 188
    inoculation 91, 108, 173
    treatment of the insane 117
    renewed interest in 167
    teaching by Company surgeons 179
    westernization, with English the official language 199
    few remaining vernacular schools 200
    status increasing with rising nationalism 225

debates on integration with modern medicine 227
disputes within Indian Medicine 228
Chopra Committee recommends integration 228
official support at Independence 231
training and research 232-3
relation to modern medicine 234
see also Indian Medicine, Unani

Babur 6, 41 (f.n.l)
Balfour, Francis 135
Bannerman, William and Helen 221
Bantam (Java) 2, 29, 30, 34, 52, 96, 107, 243
banyan (banian) 43, 50, 103, 104, 122, 127, 129
    banyan 'days' 50
    banyan 'fights' 103
Barber-Surgeons 20, 116
barbering 20, 21
    see also champinge
barbiers *see* beriberi
bark *see* Peruvian Bark, quinine
bath-houses (hummums) 54, 55, 56, 98, 169
batta 122
Bedouin medicine 6
Benares (Varanasi) 6, 79, 149, 159
Bengal x, 101, 102, 147, 152
    trading 30, 59
    unhealthiest settlement 107
    Medical Service 124, 200
    'Rape of Bengal' 127, 143 (f.n.1)
    famine 127-8
    inoculation 174
    literature 200, 209
    homoeopathy 226
    see also Calcutta
Bentinck, Lord William 140, 151, 186, 199, 200
beriberi ('barbiers') 56, 86, 97
Bernier, Francois 70
Best, Thomas 30, 35, 243
betel 126 (f.n.17), 127, 244
bezoar 25, 95, 96, 242-3
Bhavaprakasa 14
bhisti 133
Bhore, Sir Joseph, Committee 228, 231
Bijapur 171-2

Bills of Mortality 86, 108
bleeding (blood-letting) 21, 23, 24, 53, 97, 105, 106, 122, 180
    in Ayurveda 8, 9
    Portuguese 25, 68, 249
    Indian 56, 191, 194
    Europeans bleeding Indians 60, 61, 82
    dangers in India and gradually abandoned 63, 88, 109, 131, 170, 193-4
    'indianization' 68
    in Persia 83
blistering 97, 119, 168, 178, 180, 247
blood, circulation of 7, 22, 81
bobachee 129, 133
Bombay x, 70, 103, 117, 118, 159, 199, 217, 240
    given to the Company by Charles II 77
    unhealthy 84-6
    siege 108
Bontius, Jacobus 26, 242
Boughton, Gabriel 59
brahmins 8, 26, 43, 50, 58 (f.n.10), 150, 157
    medical work 11, 24, 82, 174
    criticism of 79, 103, 111, 159, 186, 188, 207
    as inoculators and vaccinators 174-9
Bramley, J.M. 199, 200
Brett, F.H. 15 (f.n.13), 197
Brown, Dr. John 125 (f.n.12)
Browne, Dr. Samuel 239
brunonian system 108, 149
    see also Brown, Dr. John
Buddhism 11, 12, 47
bungalow 114
Burma 185, 202 (f.n.8)
    War 192, 210
Burnes, James 197-9
burning of the feet 192
Buxar, Battle of 102

Calcutta 45, 85, 102, 151, 153, 199, 204, 240
    hospitals 70, 86
    city founded by Job Charnock 78
    captured by Suruj-ud-Daulah, the 'Black Hole' 101, 125 (f.n.3)
    dangerously unhealthy 107, 137, 217
    first hospitals for Indian civilians 117

see also Bengal
Calicut 2
callenture 34
calomel (mercurous chloride) 88, 89, 106, 247-8
   see also mercury
Cambay, Gulf of 30, 55
   Prince of 95
Camoens, Luís de 41 (f.n.3)
camphor 1
canals 190, 218
cannabis (ganja) 9, 163, 244, 245-6
Canning, Lord 210, 211
canning 204
cantharides (Spanish Fly) 119
Canton 2, 99 (f.n.2), 203
   see also China
Cape of Good Hope 31, 57, 164
Caraka 6, 10, 179
cardamom 250
Carnatic 48, 127
Carpue, Joseph Constantine 173
caste 11, 44, 161, 207, 223
   influence of, on servants 104, 128-9
   on soldiers 120-1, 141, 158
cataract, couching for 10, 23, 170-1, 191, 196, 222
caustics 8, 10, 171
cautery 8, 10, 21, 61, 84, 97, 112, 166, 171, 197
   of feet for cholera 9, 25, 89
   for syphilis 92
Cawnpore 211
champinge (shampooing) 56, 169, 193
chaplains 36, 45, 64, 67, 69, 209
Charles I and II 77
Charnock, Job 45, 78
Charters (Company) 19, 77, 152, 186, 203, 209, 210
chattah *see* umbrella
chaulmoogra oil 181 (f.n.4), 222
children:
   in Ayurveda 7, 10
   Indian (low caste) 54, 157, 218
   European in India 79, 154, 204, 245
   in Britain 109
   half-caste 208-9
   see also dais, women
China 2, 11, 12, 78, 90, 93, 101, 107, 131, 147, 196, 197, 203, 221, 244
   Opium War 203
   see also Canton
China Root 1, 26, 93, 112, 241
cholera 9, 24, 25, 84, 88, 89, 157, 190, 218, 221, 224 (f.n.8), 242
   see also dysentery
Chopra, Sir Ram Nath, Committee 228
cinammon 1
cinchona *see* Peruvian bark
cinnabar (mercuric sulphide) 12, 83, 168
   see also mercury
Clark, John 116
clinical trials 139, 169, 188, 240
Clive, Lord (son of Robert) 178
---------- Robert 101, 127, 147, 148, 211, 252 (f.n.9)
clothing and uniforms 49, 64, 78, 105, 154, 191, 205
cobra stone 243, 244
Cochin Leg 93
   see also elephantiasis
coco-de-mer 96
coconut trees 85, 103
coction (suppuration) 22, 23
   see also wound healing
coffee 115, 250
Colledge, Thomas 196
Colombo 221
congee 81, 87
convalescence 163
Cornwallis, Charles 147, 153, 155, 185
Corporation of Surgeons 116, 189
couching *see* cataract
Court (of Directors) *see* Directors
cow-dung 91, 97, 156, 189, 239, 249
cow-itch 169
cow's urine 249
Cromwell 77
croton oil 187
Cruso, Thomas 172
Cunningham, Mr. 102
cupping 9, 106, 189

dacoity 143 (f.n.2)
dais (midwives) 104, 157, 218
   skill with abortions 10, 104, 209
Dalhousie, Lord 186, 204, 216

Dalton's Madhouse 163
Danish Company, The 2, 209
dates 251
datura (stramonium) 66, 246
Delhi 60, 101
-------- Boil 101, 220
dental treatment 21
   see also toothache
diabetes 9
Diamond Harbour 107
Diaz, Bartholomew 1
diet 13, 50, 63, 64, 88, 133
   in Ayurveda/Unani 6, 7, 8, 10
   in the heat 49, 65, 68, 80, 115, 132
   in hospital 118, 135, 139
   in wound healing 110
Directors, Court of ix, 59, 67, 70, 80, 109, 122, 127, 163
   founding the Company 19
   discipline 36-7, 47
   private trading 46
   supply of alcohol 52, 66
   urging peace and economy 77, 101, 118, 147, 161, 185
   urging justice to Indians 102
   requesting medical information 86, 108, 136, 162
   last day of authority 211
dispensaries 159, 197
Disraeli 211
Doctrine of Lapse 210
doolies 141, 211
doshas 7, 233
   see also humours, *kapha, pitta, vata*
Downton, Nicholas 36
dracunculus *see* Guinea Worm
Dravidians 5
dressers, Indian 118, 120, 160-1, 247
drowning 35
Duncan, Jonathan 149, 202 (f.n.1)
Dupleix, Joseph Francois 101, 126 (f.n.21)
durbar 30
Dutch Company, The ix, 1, 26, 30, 33, 35, 46, 47, 51, 53, 65, 79, 94, 197, 209, 239, 246
   established in the East Indies; defeating the English - the Massacre at Amboyna 31
   confined to the East Indies 77
   defeated by the English 102
dysentery (flux) 2, 22, 32, 34, 38, 39, 52, 63, 80, 88, 89, 109
   amoebic 90
   associated 'hepatitis' 90, 110, 248
   see also cholera

East India Company, The English/British ix, x, 2, 43, 45, 46, 47, 56, 57, 67, 70, 72, 77, 79, 101, 102, 116, 122-3, 131, 148, 153, 169
   the first Charter 19
   first expeditions (to East Indies) 29
   first factory in India (Surat) 29
   conflict with the Dutch 30
   Massacre at Amboyna 31
   Portuguese defeated in sea-battles 31
   Embassy of Sir Thomas Roe 36
   Fort St. George built 59
   Calcutta (Fort William) founded 78
   criticisms in England 78
   factory in China - establishment of the tea trade 78, 99 (f.n.2)
   increasing power - Battle of Plassey 102
   French defeated 102
   Dutch defeated 102
   Emperor under British 'protection' 102
   all settlements unhealthy 107
   'the Rape of Bengal' 127, 143 (f.n.1)
   complaints in England 142
   Parliament beginning to take over control 142, 147
   Warren Hastings as Governor-General 147
   Cornwallis' reforms 147
   Colleges for Indians 149, 151-2
   the Enlightenment - interest in Indian culture, science and medicine - orientalism 149
   Haileybury College 152
   Lord Wellesley, Governor General, continuous wars, imperialism 185
   Macaulay's 'Education Minute', English the official language 186
   Colleges and Schools to teach only western ('modern') medicine 199
   the first universities 201
   the Government of British India 203

the opium trade and war with China 203
increasing control by Parliament 203
the lead up to the Mutiny 209-11
Company held responsible, power transferred to the Crown 211
see also private trading, surgeons, voyages

East Indiamen 113, 123, 131, 134
East Indies ix, 1, 2, 29 31, 36, 48, 77, 96, 107 242, 247
Edinburgh 117
education, Indian:
   medical x, 86, 118, 161, 179-80, 199-200
   general 152, 179, 186
   change to western 180
   scientific 201
   universities 201
Education Minute (Macaulay) 186, 202 (f.n.3)
elephant 50 242, 249
elephantiasis 150, 196
   see also Cochin Leg, scrotum
Elizabeth, Queen 19
emetine *see* ipecacuanha
Enlightenment, The x, 149
Esdale, James 196
European medicine *see* western medicine
Everest, George 201
eye, diseases 1, 10, 11
   see also cataract

factor 58 (f.n.9)
famine 43, 223
   in Western India 71-3
   in Bengal 127
Farrukh, Emperor 74 (f.n.l), 101
fat, medicinal 249
Fayrer, Joseph 215, 220
fevers 22, 24, 40, 86-8, 109, 138, 156, 190
   Indian regime of cooling and abstinence 63, 80, 168, 193
   Indian resistance 68
   sol-lunar influence 135, 156
   Indian remedies 169, 243
   see also malaria
filariasis *see* Cochin Leg
Findlay, James 172
firman (permit) 31, 44

'Fishing-Fleet' 78, 209
fistula-in-ano 10, 234
flogging *see* punishment
Floris, Peter 39
flux, flixe *see* dysentery
folk-medicine ix, 3, 6, 14, 56, 57, 109, 167-8, 232, 234
Forbes, James 141, 186
Fort St. George (Madras) 53, 59, 78, 85, 86, 101, 102, 108, 240
   first Company hospital 70
Fort Marlborough (Sumatra) 101
Fort William (Calcutta) 78, 101, 107
   College 152
fractures and dislocations 5, 9, 37, 168
French Company, The ix, x, 2, 101, 102
Freyer, Sir Peter 222
Fryer, John 81-5, 240

Galen 1, 6, 13, 22, 23 63, 68, 87
Gama, Vasco da 2, 41 (f.n.3)
Gandhi, Mahatma 15 (f.n.1), 231, 233
Ganges 50, 59, 65, 88, 115, 159, 174, 192, 221, 226, 244
General Relief of Troops 155
gentoo 63
ghee 10, 133
ginger 1
ginseng 57
Goa 2, 6, 24, 25, 30, 88, 92, 243
   see also Portuguese Company
Golconda 60, 242
gold 12, 13, 27 (f.n.4)
Goodeve, Dr. H. H. 200
Grant, John, and his Committee 199, 200
Grant, Sir Robert 199
griffin 64, 160
guiacum 93
Guinea Worm (dracunculus) 94
gunpowder 23, 37
Gupta, Pandit Madhusudan 199, 200

Haffkine Institute 221
Hahnemann, Samuel 16 (f.n.15), 225
Haider Ali 127, 140
Haileybury College 152
hailstones 169

hakim, hakeem 10, 12, 188
  see also Unani
Hakluyt, Richard 19
Hall, John 48
Hamilton, William 74 (f.n.l), 101
hare-lip 9
Harvey, William 20, 57, 74 (f.n.6), 81
Hastings, Warren 147, 149, 200
Hawkins, William 29, 51
heat 48, 52, 56, 63, 64, 66, 105
  measures against 132, 154-5, 191, 192-3, 204
  ---------- stroke/apoplexy 34, 49, 100, 106, 156, 193
henna 250
hepatitis *see* dysentery
Heyne, Benjamin 240
Hippocrates 6, 13
Holwell, Joseph Zephaniah 108, 125 (f.n.3, 11), 174
home leave 123, 148, 164
homoeopathy 8, 15 (f.n.l), 16 (f.n.15), 189, 225-6
honey 10, 250
Honigberger, John Martin 194, 225
Hong Kong 203
hookah 104, 129, 205, 250
  see also tobacco
hook-swinging 158
hospitals:
  Muslim 12
  animal 12, 55
  Portuguese in Goa 25
  Company 66, 85-6, 117-8, 135, 138-9
  Indian civilian 85, 117, 157, 158-60, 161, 218 (women)
  Indian military 120, 160, 161
  on campaign 141
  Lock (venereal) 159
  special 163
  eye 196
  see also clinical trials
hospital gangrene *see* ulcers
Huggins, William 204
hummums *see* bath-houses
humours 3, 5, 6, 7, 8, 10, 11, 13, 22, 61, 81, 141, 198
  see also doshas
Hunter, Andrew 135

Hunter, Dr. John 162
Hyderabad 130, 200, 225
hydnocarpus 9, 181 (f.n.4), 222

ice 65, 134, 193
Independence 231
India 1, 2, 5, 11, 14, 43, 77, 88, 91, 127, 204, 215
  Mogul Empire founded 6
  first Company settlement 29
  Empire breaking up 101
  knowledge increasing in Europe, orientalism 149
  westernization, with English the official language 199
  Company in control of British India 203
  Indian Mutiny, end of Company rule 211
  rising nationalism 227
  Independence 231
Indian Civil Service 147, 165 (f.n.10)
indianization 68, 110
Indian Medical Service 124, 215
  founded x
  teaching western medicine 216
  public health 217-8
  research 219
  management of individual diseases 220-2
  disbanded at Indepedence 231
  see also public health
Indian Medicine ix, x, 3, 12
  compared with western (European) medicine 3, 8, 13, 14, 22, 57, 81, 149, 167, 237
  origin in the Indus Valley 5
  in the Vedas 5
  codified into Ayurveda 6
  Muslim invasions bringing Unani 10
  Ayurveda and Unani compared 10, 11, 13, 234
  decline of surgery 10
  influence of Buddhism 11
  links with Greek medicine 13
  increasingly criticized as 'stagnant' and 'unscientific' 57, 80, 111-2, 170, 186, 188, 189
  renewed interest in 149
  teaching by Company surgeons in vernaculars and English 179-80

craft operations in certain families, the 'Indian' operation 170-3
British support withdrawn 187
increasing status with growing nationalism 225
debates on integration with 'modern' 225, 227
disputes within 228
Bhore Committee 228
Chopra Committee recommends integration 228
official support after Independence 231
training and research 232
relation to 'modern' medicine 234
see also Ayurveda, folk-medicine, Naturopathy, Homoeopathy, Indian surgery, Siddha, Unani, Yoga
Indian Mutiny ix, 211
Indian National Congress 227
'Indian' operation x, 173
see also nose reconstruction
Indian Picturesque 149
Indian science 152
Indian surgery ix, 8, 9, 10, 170-2
'Indian' operation x, 173
Indus Valley Civilization 5
infanticide 150, 165 (f.n.4), 186, 218
inoculation:
by Indians 91, 108, 173
in England 109
by British in India 174-8
see also smallpox
insanity *see* mental illness
Invalid Corps 148-9, 163
ipecacuanha 90, 110, 113, 241
Islamic medicine 3, 6, 11, 14
see also Unani
Ives, Edward 240

Jackson, Dr. 123
Jahangir, Emperor 29, 43, 47, 51, 67, 91
Jai Singh II, Maharajah of Jaipur 152
jails 121, 143 (f.n.2), 151
Jains 43, 55
Jakarta 2
James I 30, 243
------- II 77
Japan 30, 92, 197

Java 2
Jenner, Edward 176
Jesuits 25, 30, 47, 197, 243, 246
Jodrell, Sir Paul 121
Johnson, Surgeon John 16 (f.n.16), 165 (f.n.10)
Jones, Sir William 149, 170, 185, 186, 187
journals: Asiatick Researches 150, 169
medical 116, 187, 188, 189, 190, 241

kala azar 270
kapha 7
karma 6
Kindersley, Mrs 111
Kipling, Rudyard 143 (f.n.7), 181 (f.n.15)
Koch, Robert 221
Koenig, John 240

Lahore 194, 225
Lan, Pitre de 60
Lancaster, James 29, 33
language 43, 103, 128, 152, 189, 207
English, the official x, 186, 199, 207
lascars 35, 138, 157
leeches 9, 56, 170, 180, 194
leprosy 9, 22, 165 (f.n.5), 168, 219, 221
life assurance in India 190
Lind, James 27 (f.n.5), 114, 115
Linschoten, Jan Huyghen van 26, 171
lithotomy (for stone in the bladder) 9, 23, 170, 191, 195, 222, 244
liver 90, 98, 134, 156, 190, 191
see also dysentery
Lucas, Colley Lyon 172
lunatic asylums *see* mental illness

Macao 196
Macaulay, Lord 186
Maclean, Dr William 200
Madhava 10
Madras x, 59, 85, 199, 217, 239
attacked by the French 101-2
unhealthy 108, 217
hospitals 117-8, 159
see also Fort St. George
Mahrattas 77, 103, 185

Malabar china 99 (f.n.9)
malaria 86-7, 114, 216, 218, 220, 223, 246
    see also fevers
Malays 129
Maldivy Coco-Nut (coco-de-mer) 96
mango 93, 133, 251
Manucci, Nicolao 60, 172
Marshall, John 61
Medical Societies 168, 189, 190, 241
melon 251
mental illness 23, 109, 117, 162-3
    in Ayurveda 7, 9
    in Unani 10, 12
    stress/psychological 2, 33, 52, 98, 131, 204
    Indian treatment 117
    lunatic asylums 159, 162
    for Indians 163
mercury 8, 14, 22, 53, 97
    ill-effects 12, 21, 63, 93, 173, 191, 192, 247
    in India 13, 14
    in fevers 88
    in dysentery and liver diseases 89, 98, 109
    specific for Indian diseases 248
    see also calomel, cinnabar
mesmerism 196
Middleton, Sir Henry 29, 34
midwives *see* dais
milk-bush 168
Mill, James 186, 211
missionaries ix, 11, 45, 85, 128, 178, 209, 218
mithradates 188
mofussil 123, 159
mongoose 95
monsoon 1, 31, 123, 131, 140, 141
Montagu, Lady Mary Wortley 109
moonshee 152
Morley-Minto reforms 227
'mort-de-chien' 27 (f.n.8), 63
    see also cholera
mosquito 87, 110, 114, 193, 218
moxibustion (with mugwort) 197
mummy (mumia) 248-9
Mundy, Peter 71
Munro, Sir Thomas 151
musk 241, 250

Mussoorie 241
mutiny 46, 121, 130, 132
    see also Indian Mutiny
Mysore 127, 185
    Wars 127, 135, 171, 172, 181 (f.n.11)

nabob 123
nationalism, Indian x, 225, 227
Naturopathy 15 (f.n.1), 233-4
Nehru, Jawaharlal 231, 233
Netley (hospital) 211
Niebuhr, Capt. 149
North, Lord 147
nose, reconstruction of 9, 11, 171-3, 194
nux vomica *see* strychnine

Ogilvy, Surgeon 197
oiling the skin 54, 91, 168
opium 10, 21, 51, 52, 60, 88, 89, 93, 97, 110, 151, 198, 203, 205, 241, 244-5
    high usage by Indians 80, 84, 133, 158
Opium War 203
Orta, Garcia da 24, 88, 92, 239, 242
O'Shaughnessy, Sir William 204, 221, 251
Oudh 102, 210

palanquin 48, 105, 122, 129, 133, 156, 168, 169, 193, 204
Pali 15 (f.n.12)
pan, pawn *see* betel
Paracelsus 13, 21, 23
Paré, Ambroise 23, 242
Paris, Treaty of 102
Parsee 103
Pasteur Institute 220
pearl 244
pepper 1, 25, 29, 48, 77, 111, 250
Pepys, Samuel 15 (f.n.6)
Persia 2, 6, 13, 30, 48, 59, 67, 78, 82, 83, 92, 93, 94, 101, 107, 242, 245, 249
    medicine in 83-4
perspiration 154, 156
Peruvian bark ('bark') 52, 81, 88, 109, 113, 114, 115, 119, 122, 135, 139, 162, 169, 242, 246-7
    see also quinine

Pharmacopoeia, Indian 241, 251
Philip II 2, 19
physicians (English) 14, 20, 23, 81, 109, 123
pilgrims 88, 158, 218
Pillai, Ananda Ranga 120
pirates 36
pitta 5, 7
Pitt's India Bill 147
plague 22, 26, 27 (f.n.4), 54, 68, 86, 90, 219, 221, 223, 249
Plassey, Battle of 102, 211
plastic and reconstructive surgery x, 173
poisons/poisoning 7, 8, 60, 95-7, 242
pomegranate 169
Pondicherry 2, 101, 102
Poona 172
Portugal 1
Portuguese Company, The ix, 6, 14, 35, 36, 44, 46, 62, 79, 92, 137, 175, 244
    first traders in India 1
    reached Canton 2
    the 'Golden Age of Goa' 2
    Garcia da Orta in Goa, Asiatic cholera 24-5
    first European hospital in India 25
    defeated at sea by the English 30, 31
    no longer a threat 59
post-mortems 157, 193
potters, caste of 168, 170
pre-scorbutic state 32
prickly heat 105, 132
Pringle, Sir John 116
private practice 119, 121-2
------------ trading, 46, 78, 122-3, 148, 216
prostitution 92, 93
public health:
    in England 86, 136, 190-1, 217
    in India: unhealthy settlements 85, 107-8
    following English pattern 86, 108, 136-9, 150, 190-1, 217-8, 222, 228, 231-2
    see also quarantine, smallpox, water supply
pulse lore 13, 16 (f.n.16), 24
punch 155
punishment 46, 140, 151
Punjab 185, 210
purdah 104, 218
Pyrard de Laval 25
Pythagoras 13

quacks 14, 23, 60, 109, 188, 243, 248
quarantine 70, 136, 137, 190
quinine 52, 81, 88, 194, 198, 246, 252 (f.n.12)
    see also Peruvian bark

rabies 97, 220
Rajputs 245
Rangoon 185, 192
Ranjit Singh 225
rats 91
Rennell, James 107, 201
Rhazes 6
Rheede, Henrik van 239
rheumatism 191
Rhijne, Willem Ten 197
rhinoceros 96
rhubarb 1
rice 65
------- Christians 209
------- water *see* congee
Roe, Sir Thomas 30, 44, 47, 48, 51, 243
Rogers, Sir Leonard 99 (f.n.12), 219, 220, 221, 222
Ross, Major Ronald 216, 220
Roxburgh, William 139, 240
Royal College of Surgeons 189, 216
Royal Society, The 99 (f.n.5), 109, 125 (f.n.11), 239
Royle, J. F. 241, 251
Russell, Patrick 220, 240

Saharanpur 241
St. Helena 31, 36, 101
St. Thomas 93, 108
sallow-water 67
'salting' (seasoning newcomers) 70, 87, 131
saltpetre 133
Sanitary Act (1869) 217
Sanskrit 3, 5, 15, 149, 150, 199
sarsaparilla 1, 93
Saris, John 30
Scotland 117, 202 (f.n.7)
scorpion bite 95
scrotum 93, 196
    see also Cochin Leg
scurvy 2, 52, 82, 86, 97, 98, 109, 131, 135, 202, 248

Woodall prescribes fresh fruit 22
   at sea 31-4
   on land 32
   in India 116, 133, 192
   Lind's experiments 113-4
---------- grass 32
seasons (related to disease) 7, 10, 11, 69, 71, 83, 84, 153
sepoys *see* soldiers
Seringapatam 185
servants, Indian 104, 128-9, 207
sesamum oil 168
Shah Jehan, Emperor 59, 67, 77
sharks 38, 113
shrub 135
sickle-cell anaemia 74 (f.n.5)
Siddha 5, 12, 234
Sikh Wars 185, 210
Silvester, Sir John 116
Sind 185
Sircar, Mahendra Lal 219, 226
Sitala Mata 6, 178
   see also smallpox
smallpox 6, 22, 109, 110, 136, 173-9
   see also inoculation, vaccination
Smith, Henry 'Jullundur' 222
Smyth, Sir Thomas 243
snake-bite 7, 8, 94-5, 139, 220
--------- stone 95, 243
Snow, John 224 (f.n.5)
soldiers:
   Company 46, 47, 59, 64, 69, 70, 105, 110, 130, 134, 141, 148, 155
   in Indian service 46, 69, 130
   Indian (sepoys) 86, 117, 120, 130, 149, 158, 160, 207-8
   Royal 102, 105, 123
sol-lunar influence on disease 135-6, 156
Spain 1, 2, 19, 26
Spanish-Fly *see* cantharides
Spice Islands 1
spices as medicines 1, 256
spice trade ix, 1, 2
spleen 191, 196
starvation, effects of 72
stone (bladder) 52
   see also lithotomy
stramonium *see* datura
stress, psychological 2, 52, 98, 131, 204

   see also mental illness
strychnine 1, 245
sugar 250
suicide 132, 165 (f.n.14)
Sumatra 2
supernatural forces in disease 3, 6, 10, 14, 22, 23, 57, 109
   see also Sitala Mata
Surat 2, 29, 31, 40, 49, 55, 62, 64, 68, 71, 72, 77, 78, 82, 84, 85, 96, 112
Surflet, Richard 24 (f.n.7)
surgeons ix, x, 3, 6, 14, 19, 61, 68, 88, 90, 122, 135, 162, 239-41, 247, 251
   recruitment and training 20, 116, 117, 148, 189
   limited knowledge of India 23
   the voyage 37, 131
   no experience of tropical diseases, learning from Indians 53, 61, 63
   employing Indians 56, 61
   varied duties, political missions 59, 82, 198, 215
   treating Indian nobles 60, 62, 63, 82, 119, 121, 130, 197
   treating poor Indians 62, 63, 119, 157-8
   first hospitals (Company servants) 70
   critical of Indian Medicine 77, 80, 82-3, 111, 170, 186, 188
   training Indian dressers 86, 118, 160
   treating Indian soldiers (sepoys) 120-1
   military/civilian service 123, 148, 215
   Bengal Medical Service, origin of Indian Medical Service 124
   new regulations, change from 'warrant' officers to commissions 147-8
   hospitals and dispensaries for Indian civilians 158-61, 197
   re-assessing Indian Medicine 167-9
   Indian surgery and the 'Indian' operation 170-3
   inoculation for smallpox 174-6
   introduction of vaccination 176-8
   teaching Indian and western medicine to Indians in English and the vernaculars 179-80
   major surgical operations 194-6
   'westernization', teaching only western ('modern') medicine in English 199-201

end of Company rule 211
continuing as Indian Medical Service 215
see also private practice, private trading
surgical instruments 9, 118, 119, 152, 161
Suruj-ud-Daulah 101
surveying 201
Susruta 6, 7, 8, 9, 10, 170-1, 179, 234
suttee 45, 150-1, 186
Swartz, C. F. 139
Sydenham, Thomas 81, 246
'sympathy of parts' 156, 195
syphilis *see* venereal diseases

tamarind 250
Tanjore 127
tape-worm 169
tartar-emetic 220
tea 55, 115, 131, 250
---- trade 99 (f.n.2), 147, 203, 250
tetanus (lock-jaw) 97
thalassaemia 74 (f.n.5)
thorn-apple (datura) 246
tiffin 133
tikadar 174
Tippoo Singh 127, 171, 172, 185
tobacco 26, 35, 104, 114, 126 (f.n.17), 127, 156, 203, 205, 244, 249-50
see also hookah
toddy 52, 66
toothache 244
see also dental treatment
'treating' metals 12
tuberculosis 192, 232
turmeric 189
turtles 38, 113
Tytler, Dr. John 180

ulcers (hospital gangrene) 139, 140, 151
umbrella (chattah) 25, 105, 132, 156
Unani ix, 3, 6, 11, 24, 121, 194, 225, 233
compared to European medicine 3, 13, 14, 63, 167
expertise in diseases of the eye and mental disorders 11
compared to Ayurveda 11
first hospitals in India 12
decline 12, 14, 167

criticism of 80, 81, 112, 186
in Persia 83-4
renewed interest and teaching by Company surgeons 179
westernization, with English the official language 199
Hyderabad one of the few remaining vernacular schools 200
status increasing with rising nationalism 225
debates on integration with modern medicine 227
disputes within Indian Medicine 228
Chopra Committee recommends integration 228
official support at Independence 231
training and research 232-3
relation to modern medicine 234
see also Ayurveda, Indian Medicine, Islamic medicine
Underwood, John 159
universities in India 201, 219, 231
Urdu 207

vaccination 121, 159, 173, 176-9, 192, 194, 199, 222
see also smallpox
Vagbhata 10
vaidya (baid, vaid) 8
see also Ayurveda
vata 5, 7
Vedas 5, 91
Vedic Aryans 5
venereal diseases 1, 39, 97, 118, 121, 122, 139, 159
in India 8, 14, 55, 92
in Europe 22, 23
in Persia 84
special hospitals in India 92
Indian treatment 112
see also mercury
Victoria, Queen 211
voyages 20-32, 113, 116, 131, 203, 215
diseases at sea 2, 31-6
ill-health before boarding 32
surgeons 37
food and water 38, 113, 131
alcohol 39, 131
hazards on shore 31, 39, 92, 114

Waring. E. J. 251
water, drinking 38, 50, 65, 84, 108, 115, 133, 137
   at sea 38, 113, 131
   Thames and Ganges compared 39, 50
   see also ice
-------- public supply 108, 137, 157, 190, 217
   see also public health
Wateson, George 26
Wellesley, Arthur (Duke of Wellington) 185
--------, Lord 151, 185, 202 (f.n.1)
West Indies 26
western (European) medicine ix, x, 12, 81
   compared with Indian Medicine 3, 5, 13, 14, 22, 57
   in England 86, 108, 136, 189, 217
   inoculation for smallpox 173
   vaccination 176
   public health measures 190
wet-nurses 157, 245
Wilkins, Sir Charles 149
Wilson, H. H. 168
Wise, Thomas 188
women 22, 83
   in Ayurveda 7, 10
   cohabitation with Indian women 47, 79, 153, 208-9
   Indian women: low caste 54, 157, 218
   high caste 54, 104, 121, 218
   European women in India 78, 102, 111, 153-4, 156, 245
   see also children, dais, 'fishing-fleet', suttee
Wood, Charles (Lord Halifax) 201
Woodall, John 20, 23, 34, 93
wound-healing 22, 23, 33, 64, 110, 158
   see also coction
writer 58 (f.n.9)

Yoga 15 (f.n.1), 233
yogis 13, 45

zemindar 152
zenana 104

Printed in the United Kingdom
by Lightning Source UK Ltd.
130128UK00002B/40-87/A